HISTORY OF OPHTHALMOLOGY 3

ACADEMIA OPHTHALMOLOGICA INTERNATIONALIS

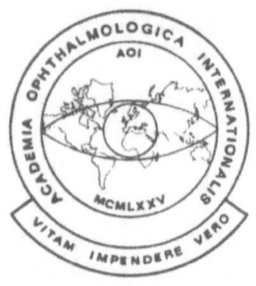

History of Ophthalmology 3

Sub auspiciis
Academiae Ophthalmologicae Internationalis

Editor H.E. HENKES
Geervliet, The Netherlands

Associate Editor Cl. ZRENNER
Tübingen, F.R.G.

Kluwer Academic Publishers

DORDRECHT / BOSTON / LONDON

ISBN-13:978-0-7923-0826-3

Published by Kluwer Academic Publishers,
P.O. Box 17, 3300 AA Dordrecht, The Netherlands.

Kluwer Academic Publishers incorporates the publishing programmes of
D. Reidel, Martinus Nijhoff, Dr W. Junk and MTP Press.

Sold and distributed in the U.S.A. and Canada
by Kluwer Academic Publishers,
101 Philip Drive, Norwell, MA 02061, U.S.A.

In all other countries, sold and distributed
by Kluwer Academic Publishers Group,
P.O. Box 322, 3300 AH Dordrecht, The Netherlands.

History of Ophthalmology, Volume 3
Reprinted from *Documenta Ophthalmologica*, Vol. 74, Nos. 1–2 (1990).

ISBN-13:978-0-7923-0826-3   e-ISBN-13:978-94-009-0641-9
DOI: 10.1007/978-94-009-0641-9

Documenta Ophthalmologica **74**: 1–8, 1990.
© 1990 *Kluwer Academic Publishers.*

Osler and ophthalmology

CHARLES H. BARNES
Department of Ophthalmology & Visual Sciences, Texas Tech University Health Sciences Center, 6th and Flint, Lubbock, TX 79430, USA

Sir William Osler (1849–1919) has been called the father of American medicine (Fig. 1). This Canadian from Dundas, Ontario is remembered as a great clinician, scientist and teacher*. His name survives as a burden for medical students and forgetful clinicians who must distinguish between the Osler-Weber-Rendu disease, the Osler-Vasquez disease, the Osler phenomenon, the Osler sign, Osler's triad, and of course Osler's nodes. Nevertheless, his most enduring contributions probably lie in the structures he imposed on medical education and medical practice. He was an active, but gentle reformer with an abiding affection for medical students and for the common physician engaged in general practice. He was instrumental in organizing a system where American medical students would first obtain a general education before going to medical school. He also changed the nature of the medical curriculum to include significant clinical experience – allowing students to actually examine and care for patients on the wards. To his credit, the institutions which he established in medical education have survived largely unchanged to the present day. In addition, he wrote *The Principles and Practice of Medicine* (1892) a seminal textbook that served as the standard reference for generations of physicians. Nevertheless, before he had done any of these things, the young Willie Osler had different plans.

The year was 1872, and Osler had just completed his medical degree at McGill University in Montreal. Like many of the medical students in the generations that would follow, Osler had a big decision to make – he had to choose a specialty. However, this was probably quite unlike most of his peers who simply assumed they would take up general practice. In fact, in Osler's day the very idea of specialization was rather vague and controversial. To be sure, many physicians tended to limit the scope of their practice to a specific area, or set of procedures, and journals were beginning to

---

*Osler taught at McGill University (Montreal), at the University of Pennsylvania and at Johns Hopkins. He was the first professor of medicine and chief physician at Johns Hopkins Hospital, Baltimore (1889–1904).   (Editor's note)

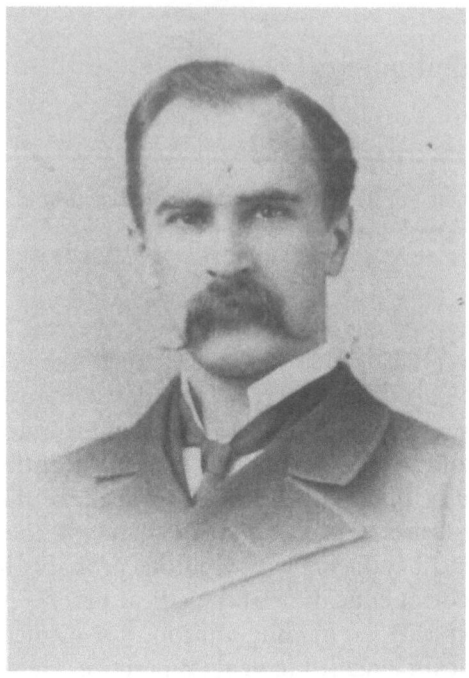

Fig. 1. William Osler, 1881 (R. Palmer Howard Collection).

appear which were limited to particular disciplines. Nevertheless, little formal organization existed among these early specialists, and there were no formal standards for their training. It was perhaps for these reasons that young Osler was attracted to ophthalmology, which was already emerging as a distinct discipline requiring specific skills and training. Periodic congresses on ophthalmology had been organized; journals were regularly published, several institutions had been founded devoted exclusively to diseases of the eye and a society dedicated to this speciality, the American Ophthalmological Society, had been founded in 1864.

Indeed, the previous 20 years had been a time of remarkable progress in ophthalmology, beginning with the invention of the ophthalmoscope by Helmholtz in 1851. It is unclear whether Osler had ever seen an ophthalmoscope – much less used one, but if he had it probably was very similar to the one designed by Anagnostakis[1], except perhaps for the addition of a small hinged frame on the back which could hold a lens to magnify the image of the fundus.[2]

The period had also been marked by significant advances in ophthalmic surgery such as the first operation for esotropia performed by Johann Friedrich Dieffenbach in 1839.[3]

Other advances from the period include Albrecht von Graefe's modified linear extraction of cataract[4] and the advent of corneal sutures – described in 1872 by Henry Willard Williams', a Boston ophthalmologist.[5] However, it is doubtful Osler had heard much about this for it was regarded as a solution without a problem by Williams contemporaries, who simply placed corneal incisions in apposition following cataract extraction, bandaged the eye for weeks and allowed it to heal itself.[6]

Thus it appears that Osler had chosen ophthalmology at a time when it offered new and exciting diagnostic and therapeutic modalities. Yet one may still ask what his personal objectives were – what sort of life did he envision as an ophthalmic surgeon?

Harvey Cushing, in his massive biography of Osler states, he 'decided on a specialty which would permit him in his spare hours to pursue science rather than to have practice pursue him, as would be the case were he to succeed as a general practitioner.'[7] It is unclear why Cushing believed Osler planned to pursue science in his free time. This perhaps could be inferred from Osler's demonstrated interest in physiology and pathology. Also, there had already been talk of him returning to McGill as a member of the faculty. However, Osler himself did not cloak his goals in such lofty ideals. After he abandoned the project he wrote to R. Palmer Howard, his mentor at McGill University, and stated:

I had hoped in an ophthalmic practice to have a considerable amount of time at my disposal, and a fair return in a shorter time, but in a general practice which will be much slower to obtain (if it becomes of any size) whatever time you have is always liable to be broken in upon.[8]

He continues in the letter to state he 'wants something definite stated as regards [his] future connection with McGill College,' because it simply would not pay for him to continue studying physiology without an assurance.[9]

Nevertheless, one can hardly fault young Osler for wanting a secure and comfortable life. He was certainly not the last student doctor to choose a specialty in hopes of having lots of free time and money, and in fairness, many physicians in general practice in his day had a rather meager income. In the same letter, Osler goes on to state that the recollection of his early mentor Dr. James Bovell who 'tried to work at Physiology and Practice both, and failed at both was too green in [his] memory to allow him to take any other course'[10] In addition, Osler was painfully dependent on his family for financial support and would remain so for several years after taking up general practice. No doubt the anticipation of this was uncomfortable for the young man. However, one can of course question Osler's assessment of the demands of ophthalmic practice. There were no ophthalmologists in Montreal at that time, and it is unclear whether Osler had ever actually met one before presenting himself at Moorfields for training under the most eminent ophthalmologist of the time – Sir William Bowman. However, if he had asked Bowman about the free time of ophthalmologists he would have certainly come away with a different perspective, because ophthalmology had dogged that great man. He had been trained as a general surgeon, and would have preferred to remain a general surgeon, but he was cursed with such an aptitude for ocular surgery that his peers overwhelmed his practice with referrals.[11] Bowman might have also told him about his good friend Albrecht von Graefe, recently dead of consumption at age 42, who had practiced only 20 short years attending clinic daily, including Sundays, holidays, and four evenings a week, completing rounds on his hospitalized patients after midnight each day, and lecturing three times a week.[12]

Perhaps, young Osler did ask Bowman about the life of an ophthalmologist. Whatever transpired between them – Bowman was not sufficiently impressed to accept him for training at Moorfields. The whole episode seems rather remarkable by today's standard, for it appears that Osler packed his belongings, purchased his passage, and went to England for the stated purpose of studying under Bowman without having ever corresponded with him. However, the whole episode occurred during an extended period of travel and study abroad. Such a *Wanderjahr* was the culmination of a young man's education in the nineteenth century. While it appears that some discussion of ophthalmology must have transpired between Osler and Howard prior to his leaving Canada, it is also clear that Osler was out for an adventure, and was willing to accept whatever academic opportunities Europe might have to offer.

As for Bowman, it appears that he did not simply reject young Osler out of hand. Cushing reports that Bowman 'advised the young man, whatever he was to do in the future, to begin with a period of work at University College Hospital with John Burdon Sanderson.'[13] Perhaps Bowman even recommended Osler to Sanderson, for he did indeed go on to spend fifteen months in Sanderson's lab studying physiology. This appears to have been a postponement, rather than an abandonment of ophthalmology by Osler.

Meanwhile, the position of House Surgeon at Moorfields had been given to another Canadian named Frank Buller. One can hardly fault Bowman and the other staff at Moorfields for choosing Buller over Osler. He had spent a year in general practice, had studied ophthalmology under von Graefe in Berlin prior to his death, had studied pathology under Virchow, and physiologic optics under Helmholtz. and was a new member of the

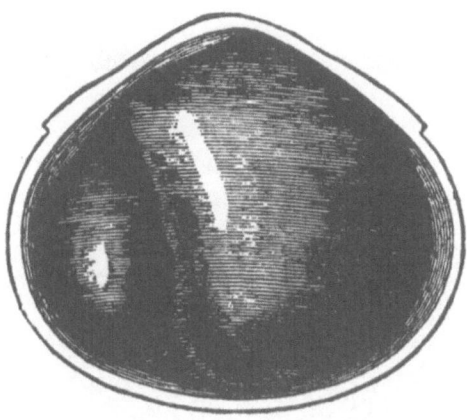

Fig. 2. Right eye (A. Proudfoot, Canadian Medical Surgical Journal IV: 297, 1875).

Royal College of Surgeons.[14] As capable a student as Osler had been, he simply did not have credentials that were comparable to Buller's.

The final blow to Osler's ophthalmic aspirations appear to have been a letter from Howard in October 1872 which stated that several trained ophthalmologists including Buller had expressed an interest in joining the staff at McGill.[15] While he expressed keen disappointment at his abandonment of ophthalmology, it is clear that returning to Montreal in any capacity was more important to Osler than the prospect of practicing ophthalmology somewhere else. Howard advised him to 'cultivate the whole field of Med. and Surg. paying especial attention to practical physiology.'[16] It is quite clear that Osler took this advice to heart from his remarkable career that literally defined the content of modern medical education and practice.

As for Buller, he did go on to practice in Montreal, and in fact shared a house with Osler. The two became friends and probably collaborated on the pathologic findings in a case report on xanthelasma presented by Buller to the Medico-Chirurgical Society in Montreal in 1879.[17] While Osler is not specifically mentioned in the report, it is quite likely that he prepared the pathologic specimens and assisted in their interpretation, since he was the only pathologist at the Montreal General Hospital and literally slept above Buller's office. It appears that Osler maintained a certain interest in ophthalmology throughout his career. He published at least two case reports – one on 'melano-sarcoma of the choroid' with A. Proudfoot,[18] (Fig. 2) and the other on a 'Case of glioma of both retinae' with G.E. Fenwick[19] (Fig. 3) and was the pathologist who examined other ophthalmic specimens reported to the Medico-Chirurgical Society. He also maintained an acquaintance with the ophthalmic community throughout his career. Many years after his

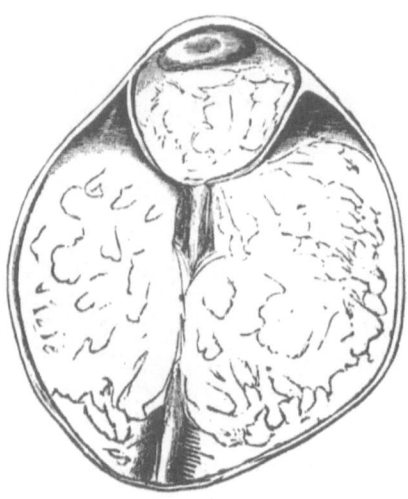

Fig. 3. Right eye (G.E. Fenwick, Canadian Medical Surgical Journal IV: 304, 1875).

death, Walter S. Atkinson, an ophthalmologist from Watertown, New York recalled his interactions with Osler in 1918 in a letter to JAMA:

> He was then Regius Professor of Medicine at Oxford, an Officer in the Canadian Army Medical Corps, and a consultant to the Duchess of Connaught Red Cross Hospital. . .
>
> On one occasion as Osler, surrounded by medical officers, was passing through a ward his sharp eyes spotted a patient with blepharospasm and marked lacrimation. He turned and asked me what treatment was being used for these men who had been gassed. I told him that in the few cases that I had seen the treatment had been mostly palliative. Osler said that if I would like to do some work on the problem he would try to have some men who had been gassed sent to me. I, of course, acquiesced and about two weeks later an ambulance train arrived filled mostly with soldiers who had been gassed within the past 48 hours.[20]

Atkinson went on to tell of Osler's assistance in meeting the London ophthalmic community and his personal advice for the young ophthalmologist which included settling in a city with a university and medical college, keeping up with the current literature, and regular attendance at medical meetings. He also suggested for the first two or three years he should listen and say very little.[21]

Whatever Osler's ongoing relationship to the ophthalmic community, it would be unfair to say that he harbored longstanding regrets over his failure to enter the specialty. Certainly it was a bitter disappointment at first, but Osler's life and career were so remarkable after that, that one can make little of the fact that he continued to interact with a number of ophthalmologists. He no doubt knew a number of specialists in all manner of disciplines and could have as easily referred a young physician to their meetings as well.

As for ophthalmology, it doubtless lost the services of an astute clinician, but probably profited more from Osler entering general practice than it ever could have from the observations he might have made as an academic ophthalmologist. This, of course, also applies to any other specialty he might have considered, because the reforms that Osler made in medical education would have been difficult for a specialist to enact. Exactly because he was a generalist, he was able to speak to the medical community as a whole, and the precedents he established in general medical education were largely incorporated into all medical specialties.

In conclusion, Osler met with uncertainty and disappointment in his attempt to become an ophthalmologist, but later succeeded in a different field in ways he could not have anticipated as a young man. This episode from his life illustrates the remarkable ability he had to adjust to his circumstances and plan a constructive response. All of medicine has profited from his responses to this early failure. His example can stand as an inspiration to young physicians who meet similar failures in this day when training in many specialties – including ophthalmology, is so competitive.

Acknowledgements

Special thanks to R. Palmer Howard, MD and Frederick C. Blodi, MD for their assistance in the preparation of this manuscript. Thanks also to the University of Minnesota Medical Library for the illustrations from Osler's papers.

Notes

1. von Haugwitz, Thilo: *The History of Optical Instruments for the Examination of the Eye, The History of Ophthalmology* Vol. 11, trans. F.C. Blodi (Bonn, Wayenborgh, 1986) p. A5.
2. Ibid., p. A5.
3. Hirschberg, Julius: *The History of Ophthalmology* Vol. 5, trans. F.C. Blodi (Bonn, Wayenborgh, 1985) pp. 318–319.
4. Duke-Elder, Stewart: *A Century of International Ophthalmology* (1857–1957), (London, Henry Kimpton, 1958) pp. 20–21.
5. Ibid., pp. 22–23.

8

6. Ibid., pp. 22–23.
7. Cushing, Harvey: *The Life of Sir William Osler* Vol. 1, (London, Oxford, 1925) p. 91.
8. Ibid., p. 94.
9. Ibid., p. 95.
10. Ibid., p. 95.
11. "Bowman, Sir William Paget," *The American Encyclopedia of Ophthalmology*, Vol. II, (Chicago, Cleveland Press, 1913) p. 1260.
12. Ullman, Egon von: Albrecht von Graefe: The Man and His Time, Am J Ophthalmol 38: 793–794, 1954.
13. Cushing, p. 91.
14. Snyder, Charles: Young Doctor Osler and the Road not Taken, Arch of Ophthalmol 73: 126, 1965.
15. Cushing, p. 94.
16. Ibid., p. 94.
17. Buller F.: a case of xanthelasma in the report of the Medico-Chirurgical Society by Oliver C. Edwards, Secretary, The Canada Medical Record 7: 163–164, Montreal, 1879.
18. Osler, Wm.: Histological Characters of the Tumour (A case of Melano-sarcoma of the Choroid, by A. Proudfoot); Canada Medical and Surgical Journal 4: 298–300, Montreal, 1875/6.
19. Osler, Wm.: Histological and general description of the tumours (Case of Glioma of both Retinae. Extirpation of Both Eyes, by G.E. Fenwick); Canada Medical and Surgical Journal 4: 306–308, Montreal, 1875/6.
20. Atkinson, Walter: An Osler Memorandum, JAMA 211: 2018, 1970.
21. Ibid., p. 2018.

Address for offprints: C.H. Barnes, Dept. of Ophthalmology & Visual Sciences, Texas Tech University, Health Sciences Ctr. 6th and Flint, Lubbock, TX 79430, USA.

Documenta Ophthalmologica **74**: 9–20, 1990.
© 1990 *Kluwer Academic Publishers.*

Life, eye disease and work of Joseph Plateau

GUY VERRIEST†

Abstract. The Belgian physicist Joseph Plateau (1801–1883) suffered from uveitis which made him blind at the age of 42 years and which has been ascribed to a previous solar retinitis. Plateau described many visual phenomena, including the persistence of visual impressions. He invented instruments which foreshadowed the cinema.

Introduction

The life and work of the Belgian physicist Joseph-Antoine-Ferdinand Plateau (1801–1883, Fig. 1) are interesting for ophthalmologists not only because this scientist was one of the important 19th century investigators in physiological optics, but also because the eye disease which made him totally blind during the second half of his long life has been ascribed to a former solar retinitis, which occurred in 1829 when Plateau volunteered to study the effects of strong light on the eye.

Life

Plateau was born in Brussels on October 14, 1801. He showed interest in the natural sciences since his earliest school years, performing amusing experiments in physics for his fellows and hunting butterflies during his holidays. He lost his mother at the age of 13 and his father one year later. His father, an artist who painted flowers, introduced him early to the Academy of Fine Arts in Brussels. After this father's death, Joseph and his two sisters Nathalie and Joséphine were brought up by their maternal uncle, the advocate Thirion. As the three children grieved because of the loss of their parents, Thirion boarded them out in Ohain near Waterloo. It was a bad choice as the next day saw the beginning of the celebrated battle of Waterloo and the children had to run away to the Soignes forest with the other inhabitants of the hamlet. However, Joseph again hunted butterflies, now amidst the cannon-shots.

When he reached the age of 16 years, the young Plateau began secondary school in the Athenaeum in Brussels. This event was to be of paramount

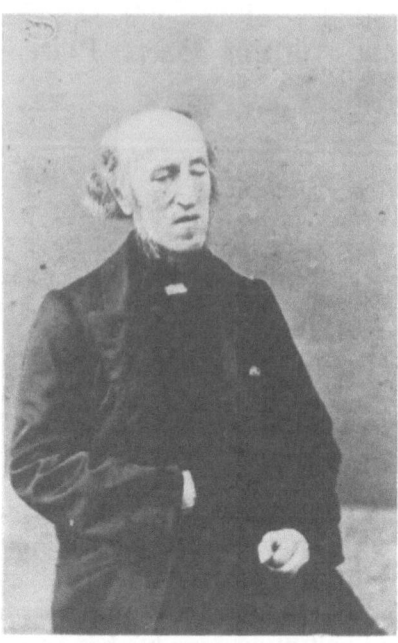

Fig. 1. Photograph of J. Plateau. From the Museum of History of Sciences in Ghent.

importance for his later career. Indeed in the Athenaeum he not only met the boys whom he entertained with juggling tricks and who remained his friends throughout his life, but also the teacher who soon became his principal guide in natural philosophy, namely Adolphe Quételet. Quételet (1796–1874) together with Galton founded the biometric and statistical sciences. After finishing secondary school in 1822, Plateau was obliged by his uncle to study law at Liège University, although he hated law. Courageously he studied science simultaneously in the same University. In 1827 his first papers appeared in Quételet's own journal 'Correspondance Mathématique et Physique'. He obtained his doctorate in physical and mathematical sciences on June 3, 1829.

During the days of the Belgian revolution against Dutch rule, his house had been occupied by Belgian volunteers who used it to shoot at the Dutch soldiers. At this time he himself was quietly living in the Ardennes, the woody southern part of Belgium. He returned to Brussels in 1830 and between 1830 and 1835 Plateau taught during the day at the Gaggia Institute and worked at night with Quételet at the Brussels observatory. He was admitted to the Royal Academy of Belgium in 1833 and afterwards published nearly all his papers in the Mémoires and the Bulletin of this society.

Again it was Quételet who advised Plateau to apply for the vacant chair of experimental physics at the University of Ghent. Plateau was nominated to the chair in Ghent University in 1835 and taught there as long as his sight permitted him to do so. We will see that Plateau became completely blind in 1843. A special royal decree conferred full emoluments on him, although he could no longer teach. After he became blind Plateau wrote as many papers as before because his mind remained keen. At the same time he was training a succession of teams of young scientists (including Léon Frédéricq, 1851–1935, founder of physiological research in Belgium) to observe the phenomena which he no longer could see himself. Plateau's later life story was that of a quiet scientist and a good family man. He died in Ghent on September 15, 1883.

Ophthalmic Disease

In 1829, like Isaac Newton many years before, Joseph Plateau performed the bold and dangerous experiment of looking directly at the sun with both eyes for more than 25 seconds. He became blind for several days. Thereafter he noticed not only a foveal scotoma, but also flashes of light in the whole visual field, while his eyes remained bloodshot for many days. In order to rest his eyes he took many walks in the countryside around Liège and Namur. Plateau himself wrote in 1882 that between 1829 and 1841 he often saw persistent brightly coloured halos around light sources.

At the end of 1841, many years after the solar retinitis occurred, Plateau suffered from the first symptoms of a disease which affected first the right and then the left eye and which resulted in his total blindness in 1843. Plateau himself and his son-in-law and biographer, G. Van der Mensbrugghe, mentioned the diagnosis of choroiditis. Jean-Pierre Nuel (1847–1920), professor of ophthalmology at Ghent University, examined Plateau's eyes when the scientist was already very old. He wrote in his obituary for Plateau (1883) that Plateau's eyes seemed to have been disturbed by a chronic iridochoroiditis. There were ciliary injection, some synechias, a cretaceous cataract, and no light perception.

Plateau himself (1882) ascribed the 1841 choroiditis and his subsequent blindness to the 1829 experiment. So also did Plateau's son-in-law Van der Mensbrugghe (1884). In fact, the whole 19th century scientific world was very much affected by this tragic story of the scholar who became blind as a result of his own experiment, and by the similarity in the destinies of Joseph Plateau, the blind visual scientist (Fig. 2), and Ludwig van Beethoven, the deaf composer. Of course, the ophthalmologist of today

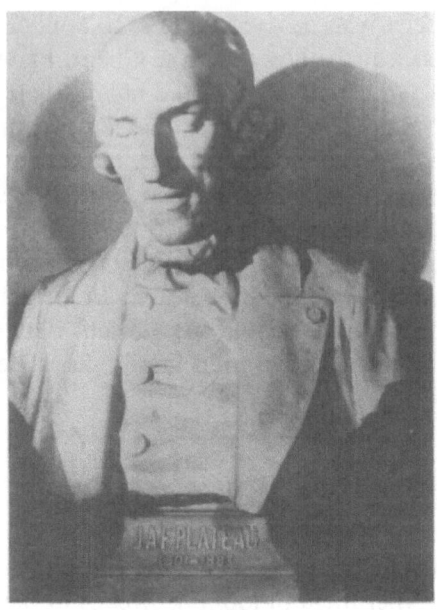

Fig. 2. Bust of J. Plateau. From the Place of the Academies in Brussels.

would probably prefer to diagnose granulomatous uveitis, with or without secondary glaucoma, as the origin of Plateau's blindness.

Plateau's contributions to physiological optics

Plateau's first paper on physiological optics 'Sur les sensations produites dans l'oeil par les différentes couleurs' ('on the sensations produced in the eye by the different colours', 1828) was a first step toward the doctoral thesis that he presented in 1829 and which was entitled 'Dissertation sur quelques propriétés des impressions produites par la lumière sur l'organe de la vue' ('Dissertation on some properties of the impressions produced by light in the organ of sight').

In this thesis, which was dedicated to Quételet, Plateau described the persistence of visual impressions very well, a phenomenon which was not well known before this time. It is through the persistence of visual impressions that we see falling rain drops as parallel lines, a vibrating violin string as a flat spindle, and a movie scene as seemingly continuous movement. Plateau showed that time is needed for the appearance and disappearance of an impression, that its decay becomes slower nearer its end, and that the

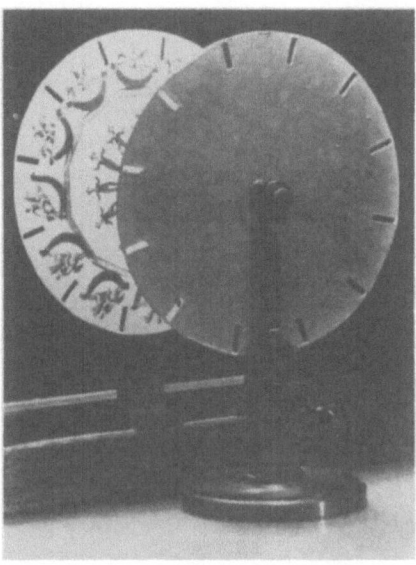

Fig. 3. Plateau's disc phenakistiscope (1832). From Verhaeghe (1960).

duration of the impression between maximal strength until near disappearance is about a third of a second.

Plateau took an important step along the path which led from the discovery of the persistence of visual impressions to cinema. In 1828, independently of Faraday, he first described how a rotating disc with radial slits at its periphery seems to be motionless when we look through the slits at the back of the rotating disc at its reflection in a mirror. Plateau's genial idea was to add to parts of Faraday's device, drawings which represented the successive phases of a movement, so that the observer perceives a moving drawing.

This astonishing discovery was soon commercialized as a toy and shamelessly copied. The first type was called a phenakistiscope and was sold both as a flat disc (Fig. 3) and as a cylindrical drum (Fig. 4). Plateau himself gave instructions to a manufacturer in London for improving an instrument called a fantascope (Fig. 5). He himself drew most of the moving figures (Fig. 6); however he was helped with one of them by Jean-Baptiste Madou (1796–1877), the best known Belgian painter and lithographer of the first half of the 19th century (Fig. 7). Plateau also constructed an instrument combining the effects of the fantascope with that of the anorthoscope, a device for obtaining anamorphosis. Several times he had to defend his prior claim to the invention of the phenakistiscope.

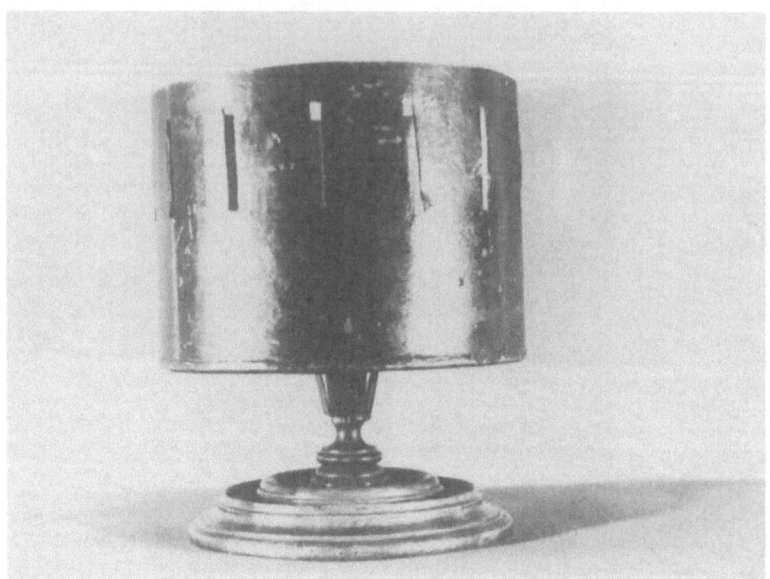

Fig. 4. So-called Plateau's zootrope. From the Museum of History of Sciences in Ghent.

Plateau was interested not only in the persistence of visual impressions, but also in all *other visual phenomena*. So, his first publication for the Royal Academy of Belgium was an 'Essai d'une théorie générale comprenant l'ensemble des apparences visuelles qui succèdent à la contemplation des objets colorés, et de celles qui accompagnent cette contemplation: c'est-à-dire la persistence des impressions sur la rétine, les couleurs accidentelles, l'irradiation, les effets de la juxtaposition des couleurs, les ombres colorées etc.' (1834). As the tital indicates, Plateau took into consideration the visual phenomena which follow stimulation, for example, the after-images, as well as those which occur simultaneously, such as simultaneous contrast phenomena. He described both very extensively and showed that the successive and simultaneous contrast effects are very similar. He investigated the successions of positive and negative after-images and even realized mixtures of the colours of images and after-images. He ascribed the contrast phenomena and the alternation to antagonistic mechanisms, the existence of which was denied by Fechner and von Helmholtz and which were only demonstrated by Hering much later. Plateau was also the first to suggest that blue and yellow are complementary colours. In a later paper published in

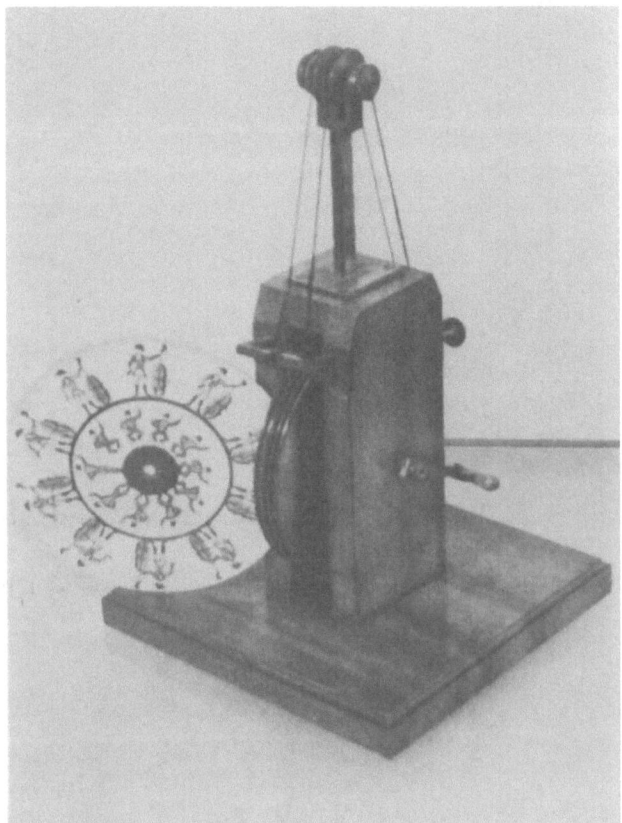

Fig. 5. Plateau's fantascope (1832). From Verhaeghe (1960).

1863, he showed that there are no effects of simultaneous colour contrast for colour strips of small angular subtense, the colour of the strip then appearing to blend with that of the background.

In the 1829 and 1834 publications already cited and more particularly in an essay published in 1839 ('Mémoire sur l'irradiation') Plateau studied very extensively the phenomenon called '*irradiation*' in French, in which a bright target on a dark background seems larger than it does on a bright background. It is by 'irradiation' that, for example, the crescent moon lit by the sun appears larger than the part lit only by the earth. Plateau constructed an instrument for measuring 'irradiation' in which the edges of two bright areas can be put visually in a straight line using a micrometer screw (Fig. 8). This instrument enabled him to show that, although its effect varies from one individual to another and from one moment to the other, 'irradiation' increases with contrast but decreases when the angular distance between two

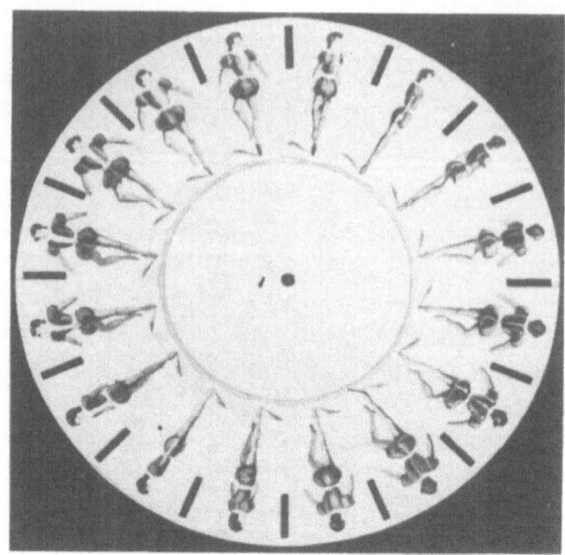

Fig. 6. Phenakistiscope disc with drawings of a dancer by J. Plateau.

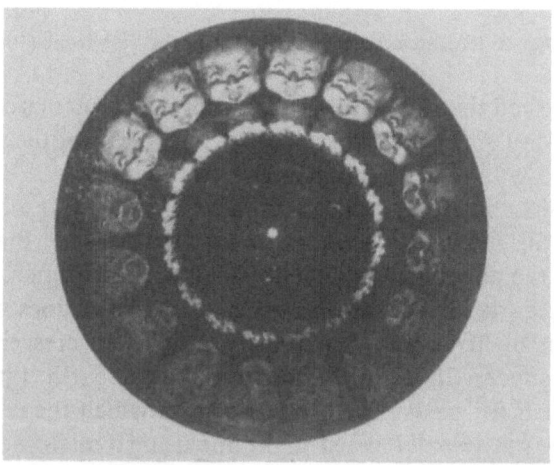

Fig. 7. Transparent fantascope disc with drawings of a blowing devil
by J.B. Madou and J. Plateau.

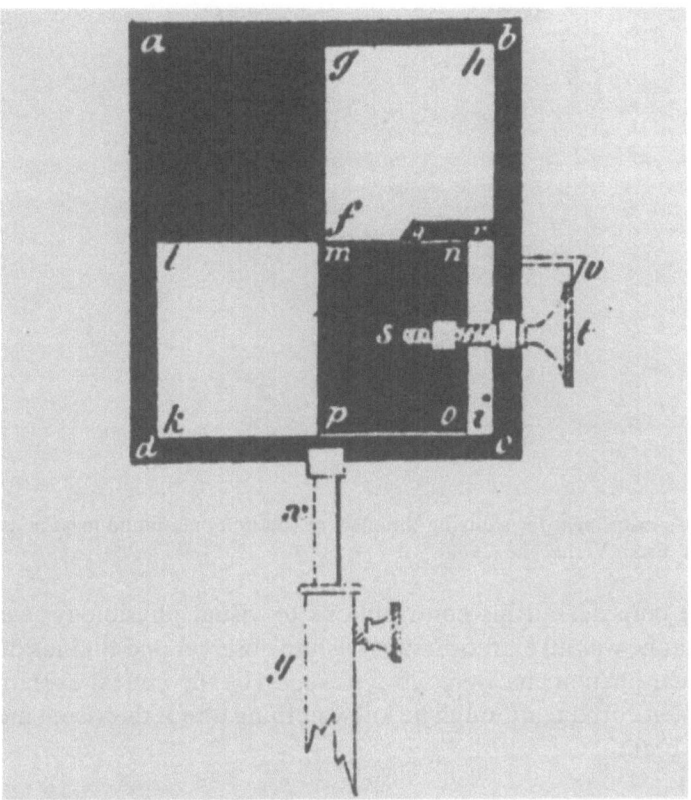

Fig. 8. Plateau's instrument for measuring 'irradiation' . From Plateau (1839).

light sources becomes very small; in fact therefore Plateau discovered Mach bands. Moreover he demonstrated that 'irradiation' is not due to the optical aberrations of the eye.

In 1872 he published a very interesting paper in which he described different means, including Talbot discs of determining the (non linear) *relationship between reflectance and lightness*. In the same paper he also considered the lightness of colour stimuli (Munsell's value, or Piéron's 'leucie'). Plateau also described the now well known optical illusion where if one looks at a rotating spiral and thereafter at a face, this face will momentarily seem to become larger or to shrink, accordingly to the direction of rotation of the spiral.

We must add that after 1877 Plateau published complete analytical and annotated lists of references (from early history) relating to all the subjective visual phenomena that he described so well. His last paper on vision (1882) concerns his sensations of vision when he was already blind.

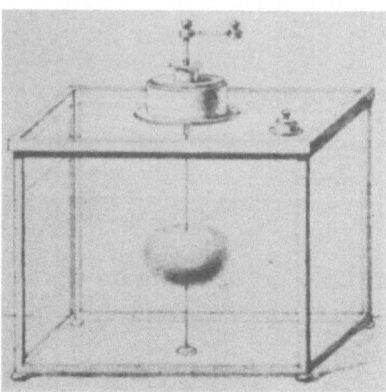

Fig. 9. Plateau's instrument for studying the effect of rotation on a liquid mass in a state of weightlessness. From Verhaeghe (1960).

When we consider all his contributions to visual physiology, we must conclude that he was an extraordinarily astute observer and that his descriptions of visual phenomena were always exact. His theoretical explanations were also often correct, although he knew nothing about the visual mechanisms of the brain.

Other scientific work

We will discuss his publications which do not concern vision briefly. The best known describes the behavior of a rotating liquid mass in a state of weightlessness when it is placed within another liquid of the same specific weight (Fig. 9). When the speed of rotation is increased, first we see a levelling of the poles, followed by the formation of a ring and the fragmentation of this ring into small rotating spheres. Plateau stressed that this experiment was not a proof of Laplace's theory on the formation of the planets, as the effects of surface tension acting in the experiment are very different from those of Newton's law of universal attraction. Plateau performed many other experiments relating to surface tension, principally by dipping metallic frames of selected geometrical shapes into soapy water (see top of Fig. 10).

In his other papers he has written about chemistry, hydrodynamics, optics (including a description of the principles of fiber optics) mathematics and analytical geometry. One of his most curious papers concerns the popular

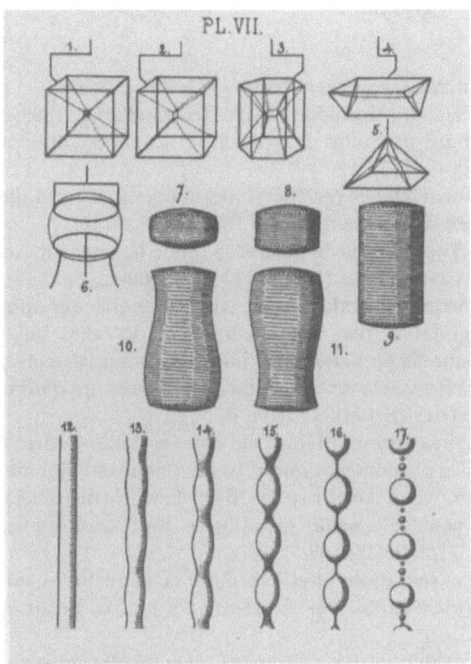

Fig. 10. Studies of J. Plateau on surface tension. From Franck (1883).

belief that Mahomet's tomb could be suspended in the air by the action of strong magnets. Plateau demonstrated mathematically that this is impossible.

Although he wrote only in French, in his time Plateau was well known outside Belgium and France. He was a member of many scientific societies, including the Institut de France in Paris, the Royal Society in London and the Academy of Sciences in Berlin.

In 1840 Joseph Plateau married Miss Augustine Clavareau, the daughter of a tax surveyor. During his honeymoon trip in Paris, he visited a famous physicist and had to confess to his wife that he forgot that he was newly married. Augustine was an exemplary spouse during the long period of her husband's blindness. She gave him three children, of whom their son Felix is worth mentioning.

Félix Plateau (1841–1910), like his father, was a member of the Royal Academy of Belgium. He became a professor of zoology and comparative anatomy at Ghent University in 1870 and in 1866 wrote a paper in which he showed that in fish and amphibians the cornea is flat because a convex anterior surface would not facilitate convergence in water.

20

References

Franck A. Jozef Plateau en zijne werken. Natura (Gent) 1888; pp. 1–17.

Nuel JP. Notice sur J. Plateau (nécrologie). Ann Oculist (Paris), 1883; 90: 150–60.

Plateau J. Sur les sensations produites dans l'oeil par les différentes couleurs. Corres Math Phys (Bruxelles), 1828; 4: 51–2.

Plateau J. Dissertation sur quelques propriétés des impressions produites par la lumière sur l'organe de la vue. Publ. H. Dessain, Liège, 1829 (in 8°, 27 p.).

Plateau J. Des illusions d'optique sur lesquelles se fonde le petit appareil appelé récemment phénakistiscope. Ann Chimie Phys (Paris), 1833; 53: 304–8.

Plateau J. Essai d'une théorie générale comprenant l'ensemble des apparences visuelles qui succèdent à la contemplation des objets colorés, et de celles qui accompagnent cette contemplation: c'est-à-dire la persistance des impressions sur la rétine, les couleurs accidentelles, l'irradiation, les effets de la juxtaposition des couleurs, les ombres colorées, etc. Mém Acad roy Sci Belles Lettres (Bruxelles) 1834; 8.

Plateau J. Mémoire sur l'irradiation. Mém Acad roy Sci Belles Lettres (Bruxelles) 1839; 11.

Plateau J. Mémoire sur les phénomènes que présente une masse liquide libre et soustraite à l'action de la pesanteur. Mém Acad roy Sci Belles Lettres (Bruxelles) 1843; 16.

Plateau J. Sur un phénomène de couleurs juxtaposées. Bull Acad roy Sci Lettres Beaux Arts Belg (Bruxelles) 1863; 31/2/16: 139–47.

Plateau J. Sur la mesure des sensations physiques et sur la loi qui lie l'intensité de ces sensations à l'intensité de la cause excitante, Bull Acad roy Sci Lettres Beaux-Arts Belg (Bruxelles) 1872; 41/2/33: 376–88.

Plateau J. Bibliographie analytique des principaux phénomènes subjectifs de la vision depuis les temps anciens jusqu'à la fin du XVIIIe siècle, suivie d'une bibliographie simple pour la partie écoulée du siècle actuel. Première section: persistance des impressions sur la rétine. Deuxième section: couleurs accidentelles ordinaires de succession. Troisième section: images qui succèdent à la contemplation d'objets brillants. Quatrième section: irradiation, 1878. Cinquième section: phénomènes ordinaires de contraste. Sixième section: ombres colorées avec supplément. Mém Acad roy Sci Belles Lettres (Bruxelles) 1877–1878; 42.

Plateau J. Deuxième supplément à la bibliographie analytique pour 1878–1879. Mém Acad roy Sci Belles Lettre (Bruxelles) 1882; 43.

Plateau J. Sur les sensations que l'auteur éprouve dans les yeux. Bull Acad roy Sci., Lettres Beaux-Arts Belg (Bruxelles) 1882; 51/3/3; 241–3.

Plateau J. Troisième supplément à la bibliographie analytique pour 1880–1881–1882. Mém Acad roy Sci Belles Lettres (Bruxelles) 1884; 45.

Van der Mensbrugghe G. Notice sur JAF Plateau. Publ. Hayez, Bruxelles, 1884 (in 8°, 98 p.).

Van der Mensbrugghe G. Joseph Plateau, pp. 54–71 in: Université de Gand, Liber Memorialis, II, publ. Vanderpoorten, Gand, 1913.

Verhaeghe J. La collection d'appareils scientifiques du physicien Joseph Plateau (1801–1883). In: Le mouvement scientifique en Belgique, 1960; 267–75.

Address for correspondence: J.J. de Laey, Dept of Ophthalmology, University Hospital, 135 De Pintelann, B-9000 Ghent, Belgium.

Documenta Ophthalmologica **74**: 21–29, 1990.

The ophthalmology of Fabricius Hildanus in the 17th century

WOLFGANG STRAUB

University of Marburg, Dept. of Ophthalmology, Marburg, FRG

Summary. Wilhelm Fabricius, born in Hilden, near Düsseldorf, (Fabricius Hildanus) lived from 1560 until 1634. He had been working as physician and surgeon in Switzerland. He left a voluminous literature posthumously edited as 'Opera observationum et curationum medicochirurgicarum'. It is a compendium of 600 extremely interesting pathological cases, some of them in form of letters to close colleagues. Ophthalmology is represented by quite a big chapter, one of them reports a successfully performed exenteratio orbitae because of a tumor. Further parts, for example, describe special ophthalmic twizzers with certain fixing mechanisms and some kind of an operation table equipped by an adjustible prop for the operator's arm. Fabricius points out that after perforation of the eye the loss of aqueous humour is not consequently noxious. He, too, demonstrates the treatment of a symblepharon and describes amongst other therapies the first successful magnetic extraction of an iron foreign body out of the eye in ophthalmic history.

Wilhelm Fabricius, known as Fabricius Hildanus, has been represented by Hirschberg (1908), the old master of opthalmic history, as a rather well-built man of pleasant appearance (Fig. 1). He latinized his native name Schmitz or Schmid – which is rather a common name still today – (smith = faber). Fabricius was born in Hilden, near Düsseldorf in 1560. In his 13th year he started studying at the Cologne Latin school. At the age of 16 he went for training to barbers at Neuss, Düsseldorf and Metz and finally to the famous Jean Griffon at Geneva where he stayed for several years. In 1586 he received a barber's licence at Lausanne. In 1587 he married Marie Collinet from Geneva. From 1591 until 1596 he studied medicine at Cologne. Then he returned to Lausanne and nearby, at Payenne, he became the town doctor. Fabricius used to travel a lot, mostly by riding on horseback. These trips were mainly done for the purpose of operating and consulting. From 1615 until 1634, when he died at Bern, he had been working as a physician and surgeon (Münchow (1983)).

Fabricius left voluminous manuscripts written in classic latin which had been edited posthumously in Frankfurt by privileges of Emperor Ferdinand III in 1646 as 'Opera observationum et curationum medico-chirurgicarum' (medical-surgical study on observations and therapies, Fig. 2). Nowadays,

22

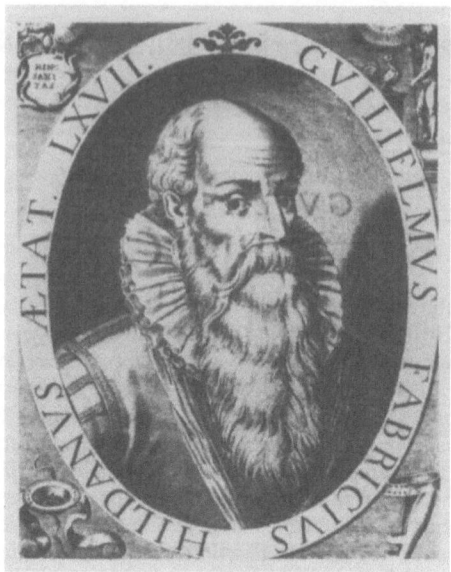

Fig. 1. Fabricius Hildanus at the age of 57 years

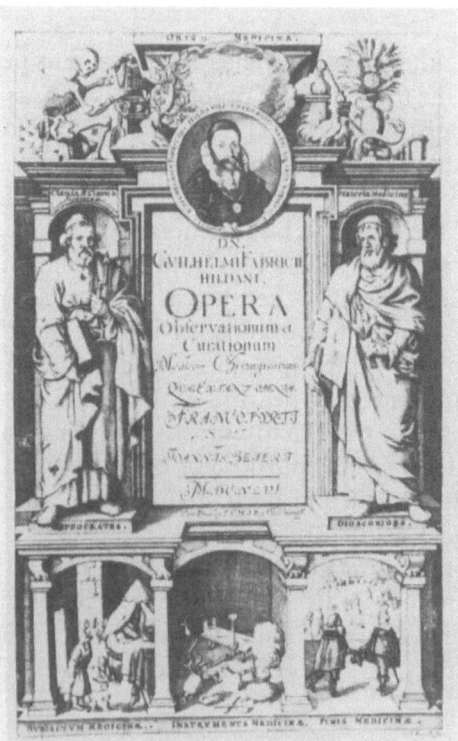

Fig. 2. Title of Fabricius Hildanus' Opera observationum et curationum medicochirurgicarum, edited in Frankfurt in 1646

it would have been a bestseller since by privilege of the French king this publication was available in France, too.

This book of 1053 pages describes 600 extremely interesting pathological cases divided into 6 groups each of which is reporting 100 observations, the 'centesimals'. Ophthalmology is represented by quite a big chapter; part of it are letters to colleagues. At the end we find the 'cista militaris', some kind of an army box, listing surgical instruments, bandages and drugs being indispensable for a doctor during the various wars of that time.

This book, indeed, is not systematically structured and only lists cases but it still contains findings which might be regarded as basic elements of modern surgery.

The first case report already presents an ophthalmological topic: An older patient (Fig. 3) showed a malignant, certainly very painful tumor protruding from the right eye. Fabricius at first tied the tumor at its base in a leather bag (Fig. 4), made an incision under the upper lid and thus removed both the tumor and the orbital masses. In fact, he performed an exenteration of the orbit. The excised material is shown in Fig. 5. The exenteration is extending to the tip of the orbit. After the operation the wound had been treated by cotton wool and bandages; the patient survived.

Another tumor extending from cornea to lacrimal gland and adhering to the upper lid had been held by special ophthalmic twizzers (Fig. 6) with

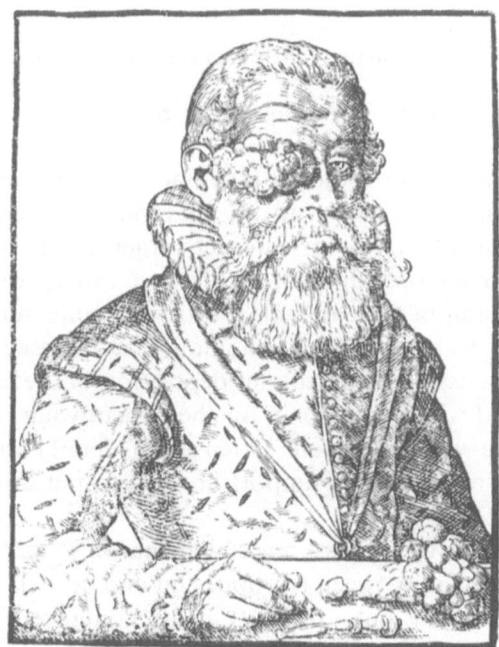

Fig. 3. Patient with malignous tumor of the right orbit

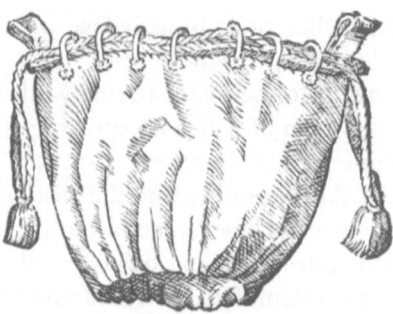

Fig. 4. Leather bag in which the tumor was wrapped before exenteration of the orbit

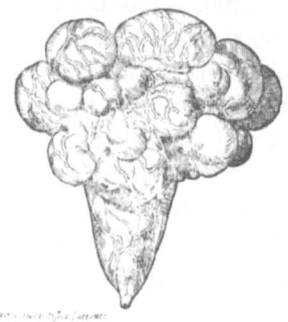

Fig. 5. The removed tumor after exenteratio orbitae

certain fixing mechanisms. The tumor was removed by a knife; healing followed.

Repeatedly, the anatomy of the eye is explained; the second centesimal of 100 cases, for instance, begins with an anatomic instruction. We find a special operating table (Fig. 7) for cataract surgery; it is equipped with an adjustable prop for the operator's arm. Also, we can see different cataract needles for depression of the cataract. Fabricius points out that after perforation of the eye the loss of aqueous humour is not consequently noxious. In one letter he discusses how in case of depression of the cataract, the eye might be perforated without any pain for the patient whilst even quite little injuries could cause very strong pain. Often and in detail Fabricius describes fistulas of the lacrimal sac. For support he used to put a hair rope in the patient's neck (Fig. 8).

After being injured by a sabre, an Italian baron (Fig. 9) happened to develop a symblepharon between left upper lid and eyeball. He was unable to open his lids. Fabricius put a probe (Fig. 10) going from the inner angle

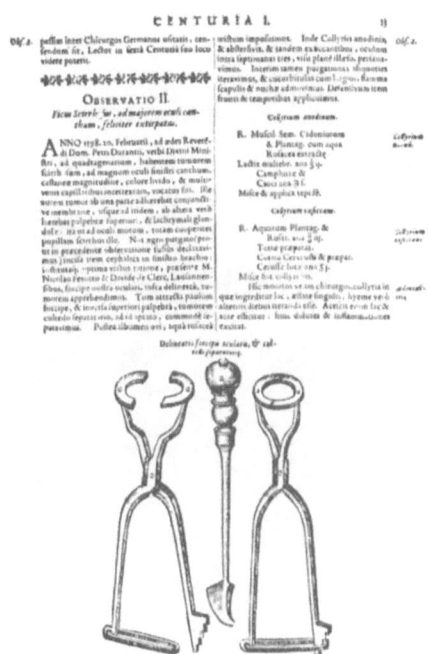

Fig. 6. Ophthalmic twizzers with fixing mechanisms

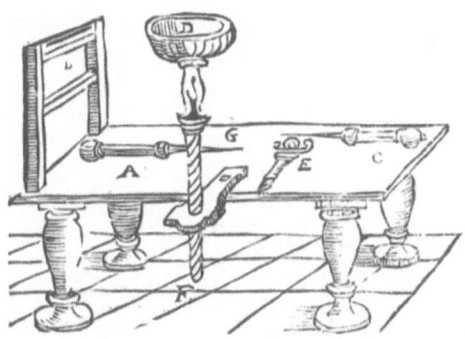

Fig. 7. Operation table with an adjustable prop for the operator's arm. On the table lie two cataract needles

of the eye through the adherences up to the outer angle, fixed a silk thread at the outer part of the probe, tore it back, tied both ends of the thread together which he finally fixed by a lead weight. One week later the adherences had separated, the eyeball remained.

34 OBSERVAT. CHIRURGIC.

Obs. 40. OBSERVATIO XL.

Setacei absq; igne adhibendi ratio.

QUum nulla sit operatio in tota Chirurgia, qua magis deterreatur æger, quæque majorem horrorem ipsi incutiat, quàm cauterium actuale, quo hactenus usi fuere Chirurgi in conficiendis setaceis: adductus sum ante annos aliquot, cogitare de comodiore & jucundiore modo applicandi illud, qui in multis cum præclaris, tum plebeis, & Coloniæ & Lausannæ ex voto successit, quique etiam hic Paterniaci Aventicorum nuper, præsente ALBERTO HAUWENEWEIGIO, Berlinensi, Medicinæ Candidato, & Chirurgicarum operationum inprimis studioso, convictore meo suavissimo, aliquoties feliciter adhibitus fuit. Eum autem modum sic administro:

Præparato satis ægro, cum victus ratione tum purgationibus, & venæ sectione, si morbus requirat & ætas permittat, tenaculam hic delineatam in promptu habeo.

Magnitudo & figura foraminum forcipis.

Hac cutem (in humili priùs scamno ægro collocato, lineaque per longitudinem colli, in medio ipsius exactè atramento ductâ, nec non utraque parte perforandâ punctis atramento itidem notatâ) quam inter secundam & tertiam, aut tertiam & quartam cervicis vertebram, à musculis separatam, digitis elevo, ministro apprehendendam, firmiterque tenendam permitto ita quidem, ut puncta atramento facta, ad forcipes foramina sint, quemadmodum monstrat figura. Obs. 40.

Deinde ab antica parte stans, pedibus meis circa patientis pedes collocatis, capiteque ejus abdomini meo, quò id (quantum fieri potest) tenere queam, imposito, forcipem sinistrâ prehendo, & dextrâ pro ferreo seu candente, adhibeo argenteum cultellum frigidum, figura hic depictæ, eumq; ancipitem & acutum, instar scalpelli quo venæ inciduntur. Hoc perforo, quod tenetur tenaculis. Mox aliâ acu, hic quoque depictâ, traduco funiculum rotundum, contextum ex serico albo aut purpureo, crassitie æquante & implente ferè ipsum foramen: longitudine quatuor spithamarum, ut circumcirca collum, & ad pectus usque propendere queat, figura autem cultelli & acus talis est.

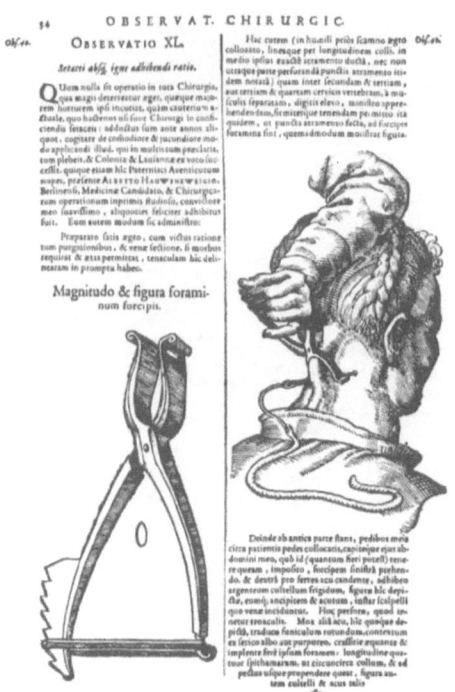

Fig. 8. Hair rope in the patient's neck used in cases of fistulas of the lacrimal sac

OBSERVATIO VII.

De Coalitione superioris palpebræ cum oculo, & quomodo separata fuerit?

COalescunt nonnunquam palpebræ vel inter se, vel cum oculo, si vulnera aut ulcera palpebrarum & oculorum negligenter curata fuerint, itaut oculus aperiri non possit, & deformitas sequatur. Hujus rei exemplum singulare

Fig. 9. Description of a symblepharon between the lift upper lid and the eye-ball

On April 25th, 1624, Fabricius wrote a letter to his friend Hagenbach (Fig. 11) telling him about his first successful magnetic extraction of an iron foreign body in ophthalmic history: According to his report (No. 21 in the 5th centesimal) a farmer intended to buy a piece of steel and tested it by beating on a hard object. A splinter sprang off and penetrated the cornea.

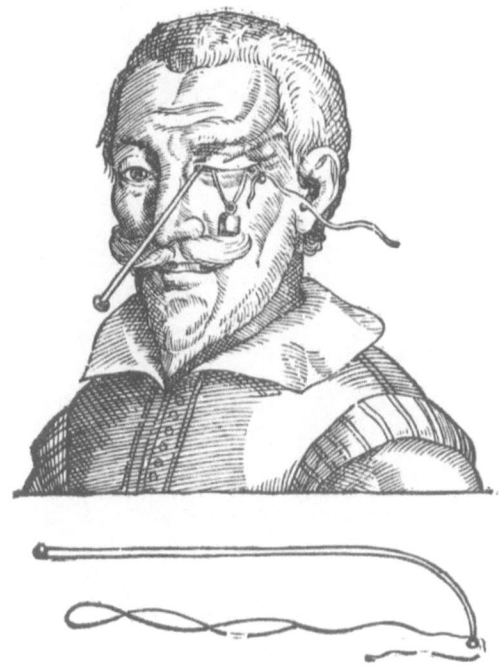

Fig. 10. Separation of the symblepharon by a silk thread

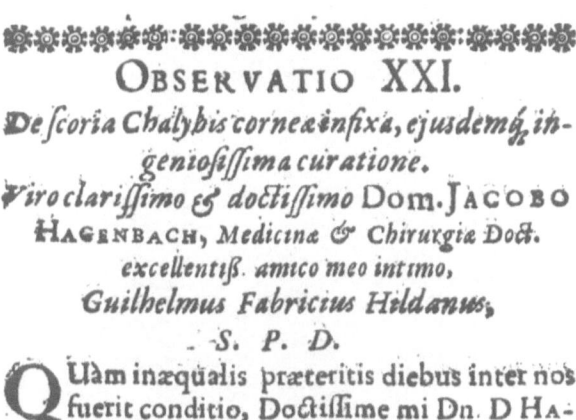

OBSERVATIO XXI.

De scoria Chalybis corneæ infixa, ejusdemꝗ, in-
geniosissima curatione.
Viro clarissimo & doctissimo Dom. JACOBO
HAGENBACH, *Medicina & Chirurgia Doct.*
excellentiß. amico meo intimo,
Guilhelmus Fabricius Hildanus,
S. P. D.

QUàm inæqualis præteritis diebus inter nos
fuerit conditio, Doctissime mi Dn. D HA-

Fig. 11. Description of the first successful magnetic extraction of an iron foreign body in ophthalmic history

For some days Fabricius tried various times to remove the splinter by instruments; but he did not succeed. Then, Mrs. Fabricius worked out a proper therapeutic procedure. Fabricius writes: "Whilst I am holding the lids open with my hands she puts the magnet as close to the patient's eye as

28

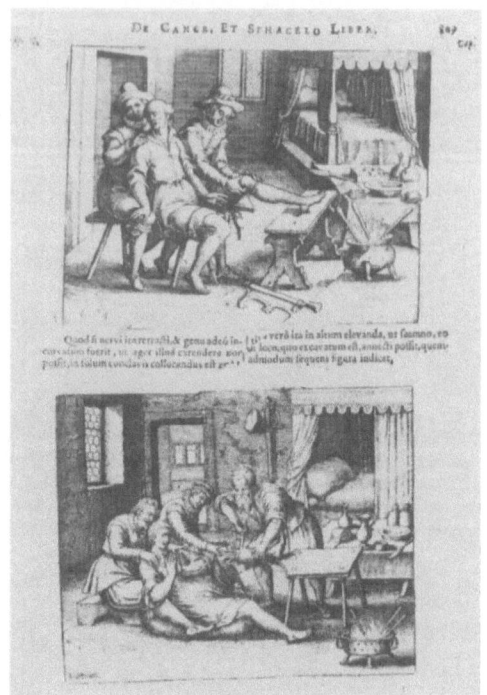

Fig. 12. Amputation of a leg

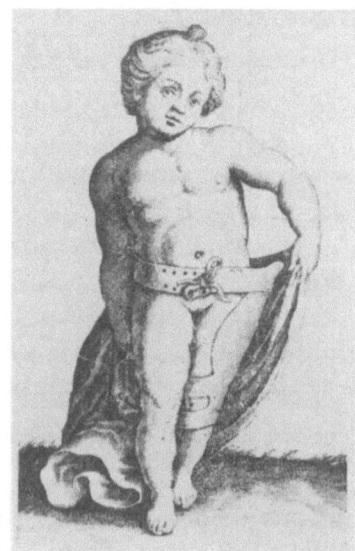

Fig. 13. Orthopedic treatment of a congenital hip-joint luxation

tolerable. Having done so repeatedly since the patient could not stand daylight which is indispensable for this procedure for a longer time, finally the splinter came off and clung to the magnet. After application of analgetic collirium, a speedy healing followed. You see, my wise and learned Hagenbach, many things are easier to be done by sensitivity and skill than by powerful actions. But anyway, you have to mind that there exists mostly contrary forces in this very magnetic piece which means that it is attracting iron at its one end and rejecting it at the other. In order to avoid mistakes one should test the sample before the operation very thoroughly so that the iron rejecting part will not approach the eye. You could master this affair quite easily in getting iron chips slowly closer and closer to the magnet." Anyhow, it is a remarkable fact that Fabricius mentions explicitly that his wife had the idea of taking a magnet.

Fabricius has presented various new findings for our specialty and furthermore he, too, has been an all-round innovative and talented surgeon. This is demonstrated at least by some illustrations of surgical operations (Fig. 12) or a bandage of a congenital hip-joint-luxation (Fig. 13).

References

Hirschberg J. Geschichte der Augenheilkunde, Kapitel XXIII, S. 353–357, in: Graefe-Saemisch Handbuch der gesamten Augenheilkunde, 2. Auflage, Bd. 13, Engelmann, Leipzig, 1908.
Münchow W. Geschichte der Augenheilkunde, S. 220–222, in Velhagen: Der Augenarzt, Bd IX, Thieme, Leipzig, 1983.

Address for correspondence: W. Straub, University of Marburg, Dept. of Ophthalmology, Marburg, FRG.

Documenta Ophthalmologica **74**: 31–35, 1990.

Ophthalmological ideas of the Byzantine author Meletius

J. LASCARATOS & M. TSIROU
Or. Taxiarchias 9, Zografou, Athens 157 72, Greece

Abstract. The authors study and analyze the ophthalmological knowledge of the monk Meletius of the Monastery of St. Trinity in Tiveriopoli, as they appear in his paper 'De Natura Hominis'. The ophthalmological knowledge of Meletius mainly concerns the anatomy and physiology of the eye. The authors reach the conclusion that Meletius' ophthalmological knowledge for the greater part is compiled from that of the ancient authors; but they define a great number of pioneering medical ideas of Meletius, of which further research could discover the origin.

Among the Byzantine authors who dealt with ophthalmology we discern two members of the clergy – Meletius the monk, from the monastery of St. Trinity in Tiveriopoli, and Nemesius, Bishop of Emesis. Both of them wrote a widescale work with the same title: 'De Natura Hominis', that have been published by some foreign authors and simultaneously – in the well-known 'Patrology' by Migne [2, 3, 4]. Of these two studies, that by Meletius is more complete, as it contains a special chapter 'About the eyes' (ch. B). According to some more recent sources Meletius was a physician and practised bleeding and cauterizing. The exact period of his life is unknown but different authors determine it somewhere between the 7th and the 13th century, most probably in the 9th. His main subjects are the anatomy and physiology of the human body, the relation between the body and the soul and the etymology of the anatomic terms. Throughout his whole work and especially in the chapter 'About the eyes' all these observations are ascertained, as well as his great admiration of the perfection of the organs, that reminds man of the Creator's wisdom and recalls his double hypostasis – of a clerical and of a physician. His study is regarded as an important historical source. He compiles at many points earlier physicians though certain moments can not be easily identified with the ideas of earlier texts. Certain scholars presume that the study is based on some unknown work of Socrates or Soranus. The question is still unsolved, but this is exactly where the value of the study lies (according to Renehan) [5]. Our own analysis is based on the 'Patrology' by Migne.

Meletius begins his study expressing his admiration of the wisdom of the Creator and consequently introduces the subjects he is going to deal with.

32

Further he dwells on the 'types of the eye', qualifying them as cool or warm, dry or wet. He characterizes wet eyes as sensitive (mentioning for example that they cannot endure smoke) but fill with tears, while dry eyes he calls insensitive, they can tolerate the exposure to smoke. He also studies the shape, the size and the colour of the eyes. Beginning the description proper Meletius mentions two optical nerves launched by the brain, before all the other nerves of the body, and points out that they differ from all the other nerves because they are 'pipe-looking and worn-out, holes that allow like tubes streaming out of optical spirit towards the eyes'. Optical nerves are carried 'to the thalamus' of the eyes, and the thalamus according to Meletius is the 'interior of the eye' where the tunics join and 'the light dwells'. Etymologically, 'thalamus' comes from 'thalpamus' (from the verb θάλπω = to make cozy). Further, optical nerves 'split in the thalamus' into thin fibres like the fibres of papyrus, that intertwine again to form a net similar to the fishing net (αμφίβληστρον, 'amphiblestron', in ancient Greek), i.e. retina. Following the retina is the second tunic raghoid (grape-like) emanating from the thin meninx that resembles a grape because of its shape (he means choroid). The outer surface of the grape-looking tunic is smooth, while the inner is hairy and spongiose, to be able to receive more veins. From the thick meninx emanates the cornea whose colour is similar to that of a horn (In Greek cornea is called 'keratoidis' (= κερατοειδής, because κέρας means horn) because it is white and consists of fibres exactly like horns. The conjunctiva is emanating 'from the membrane of the skull', according to the author. Further, the author deals with the utility of the tunics. He regards them as supporters, in particular referring to the raghoid tunic, he points out that it forms the iris from which 'optical light' is flowing out, according to the well-known doctrine of emanation of the ancient Greeks. To the same tunic he attributes different colours of the eyes. According to Renehan [5] the source of the passage that refers to the colour of the eyes, is unknown. The cornea serves for blocking the opening of the iris to prevent eye liquids from flowing outside, and in order not to impede the exit of the optical spirit, it is made of a transparent substance, exactly like in horn lanterns, that allow the emission of the light. The colour of the cornea is not 'black' as it may seem because of the underlying grape – shaped tunic, but on the contrary, it is white, which is demonstrated by the fact that it turns white when it grows thick in leucomas. According to Meletius, the liquids of the eye are three:
1) 'glass-like' (υαλῶδες, hyaloid), so-called because they look like glass (ύαλος) in colour and structure, and fill the cavity of the eyes and optical pore;
2) 'Crystal-like' liquid (crystalloid, it means the lens), so-called because of their resemblance to crystal, i.e. frozen water;

3) 'Egg-like' (ωοειδές) for their similarity to the white of an egg (aqueous humor).

The glass-like liquid serves to support and nourish the crystal-like liquid, while the egg-like prevents it from drying and simultaneously protects it from the surrounding air. That is to say, the crystal-like liquid lies between the other two and the tunics 'and this is the main part of the eye which distinguishes the surrounding objects and is the basic element of optical power'. It is obvious that the author considers the crystalloid lens to be the basic organ of sight in accordance with the well-known theories of the ancient Greeks. Afterwards Meletius deals with the functioning of the 'optical spirit', conducted from the brain to the eyes, that serves for filling the eyes and for the creation of their mass and at the same time is launched through the iris so that we can discern exterior objects 'which pass through the crystalloid', their colour, and 'brain, like a king, censures all this'. From this part one concludes that the author believes that the final processing of the irritations occurs in the brain. According to his opinion, those having a small iris from birth can see better than those with a large one (that is a correct observation) and he explains it by the fact that optical spirit rushes 'with force' through a smaller iris. Further, the author explains the reasons of the blue and black colour of the eyes and attributes the difference to the synthesis and quantity of different eye liquids. At this point the author reviews his knowledge, presented above and points out that certain particles of the eye are destined to protect the iris and expresses his admiration 'of the supreme wisdom of God'. Further he refers to the etymology of the word 'eye' and stresses that according to the poet (meaning Homer), the eyes are called 'ommata, osse, fai and opes'. The term 'Ophthalmi' (eyes) as it comes from 'οφθήναι' (ophthinae); 'fai' – because the light (φως in Greek) comes from them or they receive the light; 'ommata' – because the spirit of sight comes from them. Pupil is also called 'γληύνη' (glini) and 'ίλη' (ili), 'κρη' (cori), or 'πόρη' (chori) – 'through it spirit of sight flows'; ' λη' (ili) – from the verb 'ειλέω which means 'to surround'; – as it gives serenity to mind (γαληνούσθαι = serenity). The skin that covers the eye is called 'blepharon' (eyelid), because it has to be lifted to permit sight, and 'tarsus', because it is fleshless exactly like the tarsus (instep) of the foot in the Homeric Epics. Bristles are called 'Blefarides' (eyelashes), and they are not only ornate the eyes, but also prevent dust and other bodies from getting into them. And while all the hairs of the head grow and are cut, eyelashes don't grow purposely 'by the will of the Creator', in order not to impede the vision. Further, after dealing with the size of the eyes, the author points out that there are six eye muscles: The two that turn the eye begin from the big canthus and end in the small canthus, and the other four that move the eye directly. The first one is 'moving upwards', the second – 'downwards', the third 'to the right', the fourth 'to the left'. There is one more muscle, the seventh, which helps the eye to discern some small objects. The latter anatomic knowledge is especially impressive, because it indicates the knowledge of the existence of the ciliary muscle to which other contemporary and earlier authors do not refer; in other respects Meletius strictly follows Galen. Further he deals with vision and sums up the three main theories of the Ancients, i.e. of the Epicureans, of Aristotle and of Plato, which he derives from Galen. It is stressed that vision takes place 'straight', and through transparent media, as mainly air, clear and calm water, glass, etc. Similarly with vision, we distinguish colours, size, the shape, the place, the space, the number, the movement or the position of the objects, rough and smooth, regular and irregular, sharp and blunt. However, we discern all this by vision (sight) and feeling, as for example the fire of which we first know its shape and colour and then by sense of touch learn about its burning quality. Still sometimes vision needs confirmation by other senses in order not to make a mistake. For instance, a square tower looks round from far away and larger objects, like animals or buildings, seem mistakingly small, or an oar in the sea looks as if it were broken. Also, we have faulty vision while looking at an object through some transparent substance, especially through the mirror, and when an object moves fast. According to Meletius four conditions are required for vision to be clear: 'unhurt organ, symmetrical movement, clear air and bright light'. Also, in the same treatise in another chapter (ch. 9 'About the Face') the author mentions that the eyes are 'doubtless heralds and controllers of all the hidden secrets of the soul'. You will recognize in them 'a coward, a brave, a fallen in love, an evil-eyed, a furious, sleepy and alert, greedy and a modest character'. The chapter 'about the eyes' of Meletius' book 'De Natura Hominis' is significant because a substantial part of it is based on sources unknown till now. It must be considered beyond doubt that Meletius, as he himself admits, chooses the ideas for his thesis from different previous works. A detailed study of the text, however, reveals anatomic knowledge, that can not be easily attributed to well-known ancient Greek authors. The comparison of the retina with a net is known from Erasistratus. But comparison of its delicate texture with that of papyrus can be found in no other sources. Also, the number of tunics of the eye suggested by Meletius differs from the notion of other authors. In addition, even if the terms 'cornea' (keratoides) and 'uvea' (ragoides) as well as their etymology are well known, certain anatomic knowledge concerning thin texture of the cornea and the appearance of the vessel-saturated uvea, as mentioned above, shows that the author had in mind some original work (or a copy of it) by some distinguished ancient anatomist, perhaps, of the

Alexandrine period, because we know for sure that Meletius himself never dealt with anatomy. Apart from our own observations and those by R. Renehan, who tries to identify Meletius' sources concerning the anatomy and physiology of the eye, a comparative study of this work and of the works of ancient Greek physicians may lead to the discovery of some other similar 'original' knowledge. Our own contribution is limited to the presentation of the ophthalmological knowledge of Meletius and to pointing out certain novelties of his work because, except for some references by Gabrielides [1] this thesis did not happen to be given much attention in Greek ophthalmological literature.

References

1. Gabrielides A. On Medical knowledge and especially concerning the eye according to the Byzantine writers. Hellenic Literary Association at Constantinople. Biological committee. Meeting of the 29th November 1904; 92–102.
2. Lascaratos J. A Historical Outline of Greek ophthalmology from the Hellenistic period up to the establishment of the first universities. Bulletin of the Hellenic Ophthalmological Society, 1982; 50: 322–42.
3. Meletii Monachi. De Natura Hominis. Ch. B About the eyes. J. Migne Patrology, Paris 1860; 64: 1161–88.
4. Nemesii Episcopi Emeseni. De Natura Hominis. About Vision. J. Migne Patrology, Paris 1858; 40: 637–50.
5. Reneham R. Meletius' chapter on the eyes: An unidentified source. Symposium on Byzantine Medicine. Dumbarton Oaks Papers, 1985.

Address for correspondence: J. Lascaratos, Or. Taxiarchias 9, Zografou, Athens 157 72 Greece.

Documenta Ophthalmologica 74: 37–48, 1990.

Ophthalmology according to Aetius Amidenus

J. LASCARATOS, M. TSIROU & J. FRONIMOPOULOS
Or. Taxiarchias 9, Zografou, Athens 157 72, Greece

Abstract. The authors analyze the diseases described in the chapter 'Concerning the maladies of the eye' by the outstanding Byzantine author Aetius Amidenus. Where possible, the authors try to compare the medical ideas of Aetius with the up-to-date nosologic entities. To give a more comprehensive analysis, the authors try to complete the classification of diseases on an anatomic basis, following in most of the points that of Aetius. The ophthalmological diseases are classified as follows: a) eye-lids; b) cornea; c) sclera and conjunctiva; d) anterior chamber, iris and lens; e) lacrymal ducts; f) disturbances of the vision; and g) various others. The authors emphasize that the seventh chapter (Z' logos) constitutes a significant ophthalmologic manual, containing almost all the pertinent knowledge of that time.

Aetius, one of the most significant physicians of the Byzantine period, was born in the town of Ameda of Mesopotamia in the beginning of the 6th century. He received his medical education in Alexandria and practiced medicine first at the Byzantine Imperial Court under the title of 'Count of Opsikion'. He wrote 16 books ('Sixteen medical books' or 'tetravivlos') that contain carefully selected knowledge of previous authors as well as his own observations. Aetius dealt with pathology, surgery, gynaecology and obstetrics. Particularly, the 7th chapter of his work constitutes, to our opinion, an almost complete manual of ophthalmology, in accordance with the knowledge of his time. Only the surgical treatment of cataract is not mentioned and this omission is quite curious. Still we do not know, whether the explanation of Hirschberg, that Aetius is somehow indifferent to surgery, can be accepted, though he considers the latter a very talented writer [4]. Neuburger (1910) regards Aetius' work on ophthalmology as the best and the most extensive ancient work on our specialty [8, 9]. According to the same author, Aetius used the complete previous bibliography he knew, but added a few personal remarks, especially on therapeutics. He knows 61 eye diseases and to a certain extent foresees the anatomic basis for their classification [1, 5, 6]. Of earlier authors he cites some very important texts, mainly from Demosthenes (concerning ulcerations, abscesses, amaurosis, cataract, lagophthalmos, ectropion), from Severus (ulcerations of the eyes, foreign bodies, anthrax of the eyelids, treatment of ophthalmias of the newborn, trachoma, trichiasis, entropion) and from Antyllus (surgical treatment of entropion). In many points Aetius' work completes and widens the knowledge of Paul of Aegina. We shall attempt to analyze the chapter 'Concerning maladies of the eye', classifying anatomically the diseases. The chapter begins with the paragraph 'about the nature of the eyes', where the author remarks that treatment of the eyes varies because the organ itself i.e. the eye, is not simple but complicated, composed of tunics, liquids, and in addition is adorned with eyelids. Further, Aetius describes optical nerves and four tunics: the retina, uvea, cornea and conjunctiva; and the three liquid substances: glass-like ('yaloides' = vitreous), crystal-like ('crystalloides' = lens) or disc-like or lens-like and finally egg-like liquid (to date 'Ydatoides' or water-like aqueous humor). He continues with a brief reference to certain diseases and treatment of some of them. Subsequently he concerns himself with the importance of eye baths, prescription of wine, phlebotomy, cleansing, cauterizing and the use of some other substances as the white of an egg and of milk [1, 6, 7].

A. Diseases of eyelids

1. *Emphysema*
Aetius relying on texts by Demosthenes, calls 'emphysema' the oedema of the eye that becomes pallid, phlegmatic and itching. He remarks that it is common with elderly people, in summertime particularly, and is caused by flies' and mosquitoes' bites. Treatment involves application of honey, baths, emptying of the stomach, wine-drinking and phlebotomy.

2. *Oedema*
This disease manifests itself by swelling of the eyelids, which are heavier, less flexible and paler. It can be diagnosed by pushing the eyelid with a finger; the eyelid gives way and recovers without pain. One of the forms of oedema is scirrhous, when the eyelids become hard and puffed. It can occur along with anthrax and long-term ophthalmias.

3. *Anthrax of the eyelids*
This is, according to Severus, a certain form of phlyctaena. It appears on a strong inflammation, followed by an exaggerated heat and abundant exudation which results in formation of an eschar and swelling of the front ear: lymphatic nodes. It affects the surrounding tissues and can result in staphyloma and rupture of the eye, ankylosis of the eyelids and depilation (madarosis). It should be distinguished from sties and phymata (growths) of the eyelids.

4. *Trachoma or 'dysyma', sycosis and tylosis of the eyelids*
Aetius refers to the treatment of these diseases according to Severus. Trachoma or Dasyma, according to other authors is the appearance of the inner surface of the eyelids as harsh and covered with little milia. When the outer corners are higher, it is sycosis, because the eyelid resembles an open fig ('syco' in Greek), and if this harshness is chronic and creates callus then we talk about tylosis. A general picture is similar to that of trachoma and is cured by much collyria and scraping with iron instruments or fig leaves.

5. *Prosphysis of the lids and ankylosis*
The author discerns the prosphysis of the eyelids toward the conjunctiva (synechiae) or the cornea, or both, caused by a preceding ulceration. When the eyelids are attached to the conjunctiva, the movements of the eye are impeded, then the disease is called ankylosis. Surgical treatment of the disease is described [2].

6. *Phthiriasis of the lids*
The author observes that lice and nit can gather on the eyelids, and attributes this to voraciousness, dirtiness and a bad diet. Treatment recommended should include the removal of lice, washing with sea water and of course maintaining suitable hygiene and diet.

7. *Trichiasis of the lids – Distichiasis and Phalangosis* (by Severus)
Trichiasis is a condition where beneath the physiological eye lashes new ones grow and they prick the tunics and cause watering of the eyes. Often, the author remarks, the lids get loose and the tarsus turns inwards so that the bristles are not visible at all unless someone distends the lids. And, continues the author, 'doctors call loosening of the lids phalangosis or ptosis while they call the growth of new bristles beneath the physiological ones distichiasis'. These diseases are due to excessive dampness. Because, according to the author, '(just as) the abundance of water gives growth to plants, similarly the abundance of liquid develops the eyelashes'. Trichiasis can be cured completely only by stitching of the eyelids. In other words the author recommends surgical treatment [2], and only to those refusing it he recommends pharmaceutics. One of the pharmaceutic methods mentioned is the use of different hair-glueing substances as for instance, taurocola (a kind of natural glue), mastic and other substances which attach the hairs to the skin so that they don't get into the eyes. The author describes the method of stitching of the lids upwards and downwards according to the ancient doctor Leonidas [2].

40

8. *Ectropion* (this particular chapter originates from Demosthenes)
According to the author, ectropion occurs mostly in the lower eyelids and is caused by preceding ulceration or thickening of the lids, or sometimes by a scar which pulls the lid and deflects it outward. The author recommends surgical treatment of ectropion according to the method of Antyllus [2].

9. *Lagophthalmos* (by Demosthenes)
Lagophthalmos is a condition where the upper lid stretches up and falls open during sleep exactly as it occurs in the rabbit.* This disease may result from earlier ulcers, as in the case of anthracosis, but also from medical treatment owing to excessive stitching (iatrogenic disease). In this case the author also recommends surgery rather than pharmaceutical treatment.

10. *Ophthalmia* (by Demosthenes)
In case of ophthalmia the lids are hard and the eye itself is harder and less movable, painful, red-coloured and the patient opens the lids with difficulty after sleep.

11. *Xerophthalmia*
Xerophthalmia is a condition where the eye is dry and itching, without, however, the lids being hard.

12. *Psorophthalmia*
Psorophthalmia is a condition where the canthi are ulcerous, red and itching, the lids are red and there is a flow of salty tears.

13. *Madarosis, or tylosis*
Madarosis and tylosis are considered to be diseases of the tarsus. In case of madarosis the apoptosis of hairs is manifested, while in case of tylosis the lids become swollen and develop tyles. Consequently it is a combination of both madarosis and xerophthalmia.

14. *Abscess of the lids* (by Demosthenes)
For the abscesses of the lids the author recommends, apart from pharmaceutical treatment, which is as usual very rich, surgical treatment i.e. 'opening and squeezing of the liquid'.

15. *Lithiasis of the lids*
In this case white and harsh pores develop on the inner surface of the lids that can be seen when the lid is turned over. The treatment is surgical removal, described by the author [2].

* ('lagos' in Greek).

16. *Chalazion*
Chalazion is a condition where the lids, while inverted, show swellings which are round and transparent and resemble hail ('chalazi' in Greek). In this case the author also recommends their surgical removal [2].

17. *Sty or posthia*
Sty is the appearance of a barley-shaped swelling containing puss on the exterior surface of the lids near the eyelashes. Treatment is an easy one, involving cauterizing with a hot probe.

18. *Ganglion, atheroma, steatoma, melikirides*
These are various forms of pinguecula which the author cures by applying different medicines which cause escharosis, or by surgery.

19. *Varicosis of the lids and malignant growths*
The author regards them as malignant and incurable.

B. Diseases of cornea

1. *Ulcers*
Ulcers of the cornea can be classified in different categories [8]. *Achlys*. This refers to a superficial ulceration of the cornea which affects vision when developed in the pupil. *Nephelion* is a deeper ulcer, smaller and whiter than achlys. *Epicauma* is a superificial harsh and ash-coloured ulcer. *Eccauma* is an escharotic extensive and dirty ulcer of the cornea (or of the conjunctiva), that can result in performation of the eye and has fever origin. In this case, along with general treatment, collyria of Nile-Hiakon of Apollonius and Kleon should be administered. *Argemon* is a small ulceration by the circle of the iris. It has a white colour and half of it covers the cornea, and other half, the conjunctiva. It can become deeper and result in prolapse of the uvea. *Bothrion* is called a narrow, hollow and clean ulcer which looks like a bite. *Coeloma* is a round ulcer, deeper and wider than bothrion. In both cases a variety of collyria are also used, among them the Collyrion of Kleon and Theodosius Severus.

2. *Phlyctaena*
Phlyctaenas can affect both the conjunctiva and the lids and are divided into superficial and profound. It should be mentioned in particular that Aetius stresses that the cornea consists of four thick and strong membranes, and this remark of his, is significant in times when the microscope did not exist.

Usually phlyctaena is black if it develops under the first tunic, while it is whiter when it is under the second or the third one, because in this case it is hidden deeper in the cornea. Superficial phlyctaena can be cured easily, a deep one with more difficulty. They are very painful when they split, and in the end the patient cannot see because of the numerous scars. Finally the erosion of the cornea and ptosis of the uvea (staphyloma) can occur. To our opinion it is the first description of the bullous keratopathy.

3. *Cancerous ulcers*
According to Demosthenes, these are small, painful ulcers, with tiny varicose vessels, exuding liquid 'thin and bitter', followed by the pain in the temples and anorexia. They occur mainly in elderly people, on the ground of chronic ophthalmias and in women after climacteric. They can not be cured completely, and their treatment is paregoric. Obviously, here we have the description of chronic ulcers of the cornea [5].

4. *Malignant ulcers of the eyes.*
These are ulcers beginning sometimes from the cornea and sometimes from the conjunctiva (from the outer canthus). They manifest bad-smelling exudations, sharp pain, fever and erosion of the eye.

5. *Myokephala*
These constitute proptosis of the uvea of the size of a fly's head, caused by the erosion and rupture of the deeper ulcers of the cornea.

6. *Staphyloma*
When the cornea curves and the uvea prolapses to the size of a grape, this results in staphyloma. If the cornea does not split, the swelling looks white. However, when it splits and the choroid falls, it turns blue or black in colour.*

7. *Helos*
When the staphyloma grows bigger and is drawn out of the lid and hardens and scars appear at its base, around the cornea, squeezing it, then it is called 'Hellos' (Greek for 'nail') because it resembles the head of a nail. The return of the eye to its normal condition is impossible, though surgery can help from the aesthetic point of view. Aetius describes in detail his surgical technique [2] and other pharmaceutic treatment.

* (Staphyli = grape in Greek).

8. *Scars or leucomas*

These are white areas of the cornea, either flat or elevated, where the cornea thickens and the underlying colour becomes indistinguishable. 'Tyle covered, chronic and thick scars' can not be cured especially, when aggravated by 'glaucosis and hypochyma'. In other cases we use medicines learned from the experience of Galen. One more method of aesthetic treatment is punctuation (tattoo) of the cornea with different substances. Aetius describes the substances and the technique of tattooing which as we know, the Ancients were well aware of. As we can see this technique was developed by Ancient Greeks and was not described for the first time in the last century, by Schuh and de Wecker [2]. He also refers to the method of transforming blue pupils into black, as well as describing special treatment by Severus for the lyma of childrens' eyes.

C. Scleral and conjunctival diseases

1. *Hyposphagma*

This is caused by the rupture of the vessels of the tunics of the eye and is caused by trauma. It can be cured by great quantities of collyria containing different substances: from child's urine to the blood of a pigeon. He mentions particularly the collyria of Erasistratus, Apollonius, Memphitus and Democrites.

2. *Pterygium*

Pterygium refers to a growth or thickening of the white of the eye caused by psorophthalmia or rheumatism. Usually this growth occurs toward the big canthus and more seldomly toward the small or outer canthus. Still more rarely does it develop from the upper or the lower lid and then extend till the cornea (the latter case of pterygium from the lid is probably the description of symphysis of the lids). The author supplies many different methods of pharmaceutic treatment of pterygium, while describing at the same time the surgical approach to it [2]. Referring to the 'over-grown whites of the eye' he divides them into painful and painless. It seems that among the painless cases he includes congenital cysts, because he remarks that often bristles grow on them.

3. *Eganthis*

Eganthis the author calls the thickening of the big canthus and he notes that it occurs more often with people living by the sea. He divides eganthis into 'benign and malignant'. Apart from various therapeutic, pharmaceutic methods he suggests surgical treatment of eganthis [2].

4. *Hemorrhages of the canthi*
The author refers to hemorrages of the canthi occurring mainly in children because of constant crying and due to the stretching of anastomotic lid vessels. Obviously the case is that of bloody tears.

D. Diseases of the anterior chamber, pupil and lens

1. *Hypopyon*
In general the creation of pus in ulcers of the cornea is known as *pyosis*. *Onyhion* is pyosis when it looks like a broken nail (onyx in Greek). It corresponds to the present-day hypopyon. Hypopyon is pyosis when pus reaches the middle of the cornea or even the whole of it. It may occur, according to the author, without prior ophthalmia or ulcer. It is accompanied by erythema around the eyes and pain in the temples. Apart from general treatment consisting of clysterizing, cupping at the inion, phlebotomy, applying leeches on the temples; cauterizing is also practiced, as well as different collyria, those of Dion and Apollonius among them.

2. *Glaucosis* (by Demosthenes)
Two types of glaucosis can be distinguished. Glaucosis proper is the change of the colour toward glaucos and dryness and thickening of the crystalloid liquid. The second type is caused by preceding hypochyma.

3. *Hypochyma* (by Demosthenes)
Hypochyma is the overflow of liquids that coagulate in the pupil area. Aetius gives a complete description of the disease in the initial and advanced stages. This text by Demosthenes contains the description of the circles that patients see around the flame of lamps. This point concerning coloured circles described by Demour in the 19th century in cases of glaucomatous patients, had been described first by the ancient Greek doctor Demosthenes as we can see. We remind that hypochyma according to these descriptions is what we call today glaucoma, while glaucosis is today's cataract [8].

4. *Mydriasis or platycoria*
The meaning of mydriasis corresponds with the present meaning of the term. The author notes the impairment of vision and attributes it to disturbances of the 'optical spirit'.

5. *Phthisis of the pupil*
Phthisis of the pupil corresponds with today's *myosis* when (the pupil) becomes narrower and blunter. The author observes that patients see the

objects larger than normal size because of the narrowness of the pupil. Treatment consists of corresponding hygienic and dietary measures and of various collyria.

E. Diseases of the lacrimal ducts

1. *Aegilops* [8] (by Severus)
Aegilops is an abscess that develops near the big canthus. It is considered difficult to be cured because of its proximity to the eye. In the initial stages the treatment consists of the application of anti-inflammatory concoctions. In advanced stages cauterizing and surgical treatment are used. This case is one of chronic dacryocystitis, according to the modern meaning of the term.

2. *Anchylops* [8]
Anchylops develops in the same area as aegilops. It is painless, progresses slowly, and contains honey-like and flower liquid. Surgical treatment is used.

3. *Rhyas*
Rhyas is a condition where, due to the removal of the pterygion or eganthis, the whole canthus grows larger and swells. This results in poor drainage of tears that overflow the eyes. In other words, here we have one of the cases of epiphora. It can occur also in case of aegilops, badly treated. The disease is called rhyas, because of constant rheumatism of the eyes, accompanied with permanent flow of tears.

F. Disturbances of vision

1. *Myopia*
Myopics are called those capable from birth of seeing small objects situated near by, while they are unable to discern larg , ones from a certain distance. When reading, myopics bring the text very c iose so that 'the written matter touches the eyes'. The disease is incurable.

2. *Nyctalopia*
Nyctalopia is a condition where the patient has normal vision in daytime, at sunset he sees less and in darkness nothing at all. It may be vice versa, but much more rarely. The disease seems to be caused by some malady of the brain and mainly of the 'optical spirit', or of the liquid substances and tunics

of the eyes. Among the numerous methods of treatment that the author suggests, we point out the use of liver per os, to which he seems to attach particular significance and which seems to be quite reasonable nowadays.

3. *Amblyopia* (by Galen)
'Amblyopia is dimness of vision caused by various reasons'. The author attributes it to disturbances of the optical spirit and observes that it can also occur in cases of chronic diseases, great distress, and in elderly people.

4. *Amaurosis*
Amaurosis is 'more often complete impairment of vision without any apparent disturbance of the eyes, in other words, while the pupil seems without pathological symptoms'. The author supplies a number of general maladies that can cause this disease.

G. Other diseases

1. *Traumas*
Caused by foreign bodies (insects, hay, sand) [2].

2. *Chemical burns*
Caused by quicklime [2].

3. *Thermal burns* [2]
The author uses for treatment of these diseases different collyria, and the removal of foreign bodies. In particular, traumas are classified as bites, deeper traumas, rupture of the bulb resulting in the loss of the aqueous liquid and finally, proptosis of the eye, that can be caused by a violent hit on the head or by falling from a height (proptosis is drooping of the eye *outwards* so that it is not covered by the lids) – apparently it is the case of retrobulbar hematoma.

4. *Languor of the eyes* (by Demosthenes)
The eyes manifest languor when they cannot bear the sight of anything white, bright or blazed; watering of the eyes is caused, also and especially while reading. This disease should be distinguished from 'rhyas' because the latter causes watering of the eyes without any reason ('prophasis'). The disease can be cured by hygienic and dietary treatment.

5. *Paralysis of the eyes.* (by Demosthenes)
Apart from the optical nerve the whole eye itself or together with the lid can be paralyzed. When the whole eye is paralyzed no movement occurs. Lid

paralysis is treated by hygienic and dietary measures as well as by collyria and when that fails, surgical treatment is applied (stitching of the lid upwards). Paralysis of the eyes is difficult to cure and if it occurs from birth, it is incurable (Aetius refers to the congenital type of disease).

6. *Atrophy and phthisis of the eye*
Atrophy of the eye is a condition when the eye reduces and cannot see. It can be caused by violent headaches and sharp fever or other maladies, and is hard to cure. The difference between atrophy and phthisis is that in case of phthisis only the pupil is smaller and poorer, while in case of atrophy the whole eye is reduced.

7. *'Ecpiesmus'*
This is a condition when the eyes are drawn outward and remain in this position, as it occurs in the hanged, or athletes in extreme exhaustion, or women in labor. The author recommends phlebotomy and cleansing with some medicaments.

8. *Synchysis*
As can be seen from the description synchysis in a condition similar to atrophy, which can be often caused by the inflammation of the uvea whereupon rupture of its vessels occurs. In this case the pupil acquires a blurred colour and grows larger or smaller than normal size. This disease can also be cured by phlebotomy and different collyria. The meaning of the term differs from this in modern Greek, where it is attributed to confusion.

Aetius dedicates his last chapter to general therapeutic methods describing the arteriotomy by Severus and other methods. There are also chapters on angiology and on temple and eye compresses of Severus; on dry, liquid and sodium collyria and collyria made of incense. He also refers to the collyria of Galen, Kleon, Diagoras, Filagrius, Theodotus, Zoilus and many other ancient authors.

While analyzing the Seventh Chapter of Aetius one arrives at the conclusion that it constitutes a complete ophthalmologic manual that contains knowledge of pathology, surgery and pharmacology concerning the treatment of the eyes. It is impossible, however, while presenting this work, to refer extensively to all his pharmacological methods that are in fact rather entangled. So we limited our task to giving only a rough picture of the ophthalmological knowledge of Aetius of Ameda, and especially to interpreting different clinical pictures he unfolds, according to his own opinions and, where possible, to update his nosological conceptions. In our opinion,

48

more comprehensive presentation of his knowledge, his pharmacology and even of the surgical methods he suggests for many different ophthalmic diseases, should become subject of a separate study.

References

1. Aetii Amideni in Ed. Alexander Olivieri Libri Medicinales V–VIII. Corpus Medicorum Graecorum. Berolini in Aedibus Academiae Litterarum, 1950.
2. Anagnostakis A. Contributions à l'Histoire de la chirurgie oculaire chez les Anciens. 1872 Athènes, Perris Frères, éd.
3. Fronimopoulos, J. & Lascaratos J. Eye Injuries by the Byzantine writer Aetios Amidinos. Documenta Ophthalmologica 1988; 68: 121–9.
4. Hirschberg J. The History of Ophthalmology, Vol. I. Antiquity, Trans. F.C. Blodi, J.P. Wayenborgh. Bonn, 1982.
5. Lascaratos J & Marketos S. The eye cancer in Ancient Greece, Hellenic Oncology, 1984; 20: 44–50.
6. Lascaratos J. Ophthalmological ideas in the texts of the Byzantine writers. Byzantine Studies. 1987; Vol I'. Athens.
7. Lascaratos J & Marketos S. A historical outline of Greek ophthalmology from the Hellenistic period to the establishment of the first universities. Documenta Ophthalmologica 1988; 68: 157–69.
8. Lascaratos J & Marketos S. Ophthalmological lore in the Corpus Hippocraticum. Documenta Ophthalmologica 1988; 68: 35–45 (Glossary of ophthalmological terms in Ancient Greek texts, pp. 43–45).
9. Neuburger M. History of Medicine, Vol. I. H. Frowde, Hodder and Stoughton, London, 1910.

Address for correspondence: J. Lascaratos, Or. Taxiarchias 9, Zografou, Athens 157 72, Greece.

Documenta Ophthalmologica **74**: 49–56, 1990.

Father Waclaw Szuniewicz, M.D., an ophthalmologist of unusual courage and devotion

WITOLD J. ORLOWSKI[1], ANDRZEJ W. FRYCZKOWSKI[2] &
LECH BIEGANOWSKI[3]
[1]*Department of Ophthalmology of Karol Marcinkowski's Medical Academy in Poznan
(deceased);* [2]*The Department of Ophthalmology, Ohio State University; and* [3]*The
Ophthalmology Department, Province Hospital in Torun*

Abstract. The authors present a short biography of the missionary-priest ophthalmologist
Waclaw Szuniewicz (1892–1963). This remarkable man completed his ophthalmologic training between 1922 and 1927 at the Department of Ophthalmology of the Stefan Batory
University in Wilno, Poland. From 1931 to 1949 he served as a missionary priest in China,
and for part of this time he was the head of the Department of Ophthalmology at a hospital
in the Chinese town of Shuntehfu. He organized and ran a 100 bed ophthalmology department
there, also supervising 18 outpatient clinics in the surrounding area. During this period he
regularly saw over 145,000 patients and performed over 5000 ophthalmic operations a year!
From 1949 to 1952 Dr Szuniewicz carried out research work on the surgical treatment of
corneal astigmatism. His interesting refractive procedures were done at Yale University in the
USA and the techniques he developed arose from the work he had initially done in China from
1946 to 1948. Dr Suniewicz moved from the USA to Brazil in 1952 where he continued his
refractive surgery research until 1954 and his missionary service until his death in 1963.

Waclaw Szuniewicz (Fig. 1) was born either on December 26, 1891, or
December 28, 1892, in the small town of Glebokie (presently Glubokije) in
the Province of Wilno in Poland (under Russian partition) presently the
Belorussian SSR. He was the seventh child in his family, but only the fourth
to survive to adulthood.

Waclaw attended classical high school in Smolensk and medical school in
Moscow. He received his Medical Doctor degree from the medical school in
1916 or 1917.

Shortly after this, he was recruited into the Russian Army and served on
the Minsk Front. He served for a brief time as a staff physician at the Red
Cross Hospital in Smolensk and finally he was evacuated to the town of
Voronez located deep in Russia, where he worked in the hospital of the
Public Health Service.

After World War I, in Wilno (Poland), Dr Szuniewicz worked in the
Department of Pediatrics and in the Department of Ophthalmology at the

Stefan Batory University. Dr Szuniewicz was involved in both pediatrics and ophthalmology.

An important indirect proof of Dr Szuniewicz's ophthalmic background, is simply the fact that upon his arrival in China he was able to quickly set up and run a huge ophthalmic service. We know, for instance, that he performed glaucoma surgery such as the hemi-Elliot Szymanski procedure and the fact that when he opened the pediatric clinics he needed to bring in outside help to run them, must indicate that his primary role was that of an ophthalmologist.

The bulk of the information on his life comes from the memories of his sister Konstancja [1]. She characterized him as being cheerful and friendly, also stating that he was a quiet man who loved music, poetry, and 'everything that is beautiful'. He himself played the piano and wrote poetry.

On April 23, 1927 he started his missionary study at the Theological Seminary of the Vincent a Paulo Missionary Order in Cracow, Stradomska Str. He became priest on September 8, 1930 and read his first mass as a priest at the Missionary Church in St. Salvator's Mountain in Wilno (Poland).

In 1928, during the time of his study at the seminary, he published a paper that outlined his future plans as a missionary.

In keeping with these plans he travelled to Marseille via Paris. From there he travelled to Saigon, and next to Tjanjin (Tientcin), a northern port of China. He arrived there on January 9, 1931.

In China, he was known to the Chinese as 'Suen Wei Jen' – the man with silver barb, the highest title of respect for a physician. There he performed the roles of both priest and ophthalmologist, having a duty, as he stated, 'to treat the invisible spirit and to help people to recover sight and health.'

Dr Szuniewicz began with a small 19 bed charity hospital in Shuntehfu, a town of 80,000 residents located in the Hopeh Province of Northern China. This province consisted overall of some one million inhabitants spread over nine counties. From this small hospital Dr Szuniewicz created a 100 bed ophthalmic hospital, and up to 18 additional outpatient clinics located from 30–70 kilometers from Shuntehfu. Beginning in the autumn of 1933 he added a pediatrics service to his activities, but this started slowly and after two years there were only two outpatient pediatric clinics. Still, all of this organizational effort allowed Dr Szuniewicz to perform up to 35 surgical procedures daily, including some 800 cataract extractions per year. In addition, he examined 145,000 eye patients a year, since, as he put it, 'seldom is a Chinese family tree of trachoma; blind people are everywhere and eye disease is called the Chinese Plague.' Incidentally, Dr Szuniewicz controlled this ophthalmic empire by riding from clinic to clinic on a bicycle!

It is interesting that although he was involved in other types of medical care (i.e. pediatrics) it was important to him that the ophthalmic emphasis of his clinics and hospitals be preserved. In 1937, he wrote that, 'even in war conditions we want to continue the nature of the Ophthalmological Hospital.'

Nor was his work limited to the area around Shuntehfu. For example, at the invitation of the Apostole's delegate Archbishop Zanin, Dr Szuniewicz went to Peking where in a three month period he organized an ophthalmology ward for the Central Hospital of the Catholic University (1938).

Around 1936 the hospital in Shuntehfu was visited by the French Jesuit Father Germain, who was president of Aurora University. He wrote in the University Bulletin that, 'The fame of this Polish scientist had spread out to the surrounding provinces in Northern China. Patients came from hundreds of kilometers away to see him. His surgical procedures are recognized as extraordinary by all specialists, and that it would take ten regular physicians to do the work done by Dr Szuniewicz.' A few months later Father Germain proposed that Dr Szuniewicz collaborate with the Department of Ophthalmology at the Aurora University. He offered Dr Szuniewicz an honorary professorship and said Dr Szuniewicz's hospital could become part of the Ophthalmology Department, thereby entitling it to financial support from the university. However, Dr Szuniewicz declined the offer because he wanted to preserve the Polish character of his hospital. He had at that time two Chinese doctors training under him.

The mission there was eventually closed by the local authorities and since Dr Szuniewicz was still an effective physician and surgeon, he continued his medical missionary work elsewhere. From December, 1946 to February, 1949 he worked at the French Province Charity Nuns Hospital in Tientcin. He then worked at the French Hospital in Peking and then in two Shanghai hospitals simultaneously. He eventually decided to go to America in order to re-acquaint himself with the latest ophthalmic technology, and on Feb 6, 1949 he received his visitor's visa.

In the U.S.A., Dr Szuniewicz initially stayed with some Polish priests in Derby (in Brooklyn) before moving in October, 1949 to New Haven, Connecticut, the location of Yale University. He stayed in the house of the Vicentian Fathers in New Haven while doing research in the laboratories of Yale University. He lectured also on his extensive eye care experience in China. And all this research was in addition to his duties as priest for the St. Stanislaw parish. (Fig. 2).

On November 10, 1951 he wrote that the U.S.A. government was allowing him to begin the naturalization process. By that time, however, he had already decided to return to missionary work and had been granted a visa for Brazil. He left New York on January 24, 1952, bound for the town of

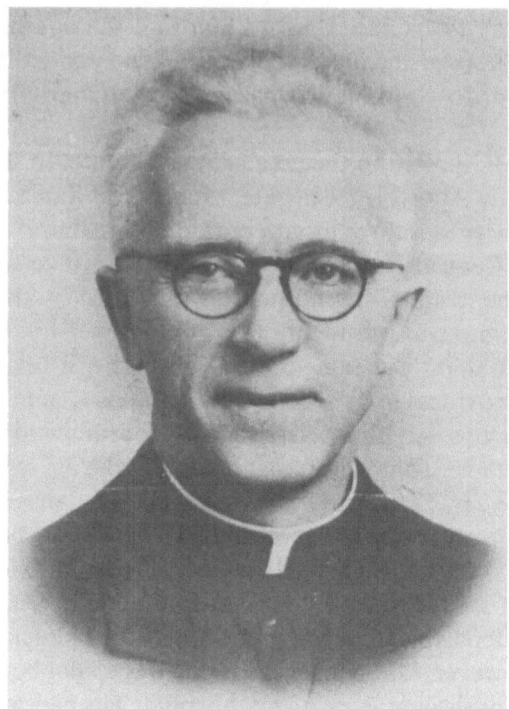

Fig. 1. Father Szuniewicz in the U.S.A.

Mafra in the Santa Catharina Province. He worked there for several years and then in June of 1956 he moved to Irati in the Parana Province where he started his parish service at the Paroquia Sao Miguel.

From Irati Dr Szuniewicz wrote, 'I have a room here that is so small I can barely fit between the table and bed. I like such small cells but what can I do when the shelves of my library and my boxes of books occupy all the free space? I cannot break off my friendship with the books, and I will probably die with a book in my hand.' From a letter dated March 4, 1957 we learn that he had about 200 volumes about China or written in Chinese alone!

During this time in Brazil he was still active as an ophthalmologist. According to the memoirs of Father Feliks Stefanowicz he was considered the 'Chinese performer of miracles.' As late as a year and a half before his death, Dr Szuniewicz wrote, 'I did not stop practicing medicine.'

Dr Szuniewicz was also an expert on languages. He spoke Polish, Russian, Latin, Chinese, English, French, and Portugese. He never forgot his Polish upbringing though. He said that, 'wherever I went I could proudly say that the Polish spirit always brought depth and kindness, belief and discovery,

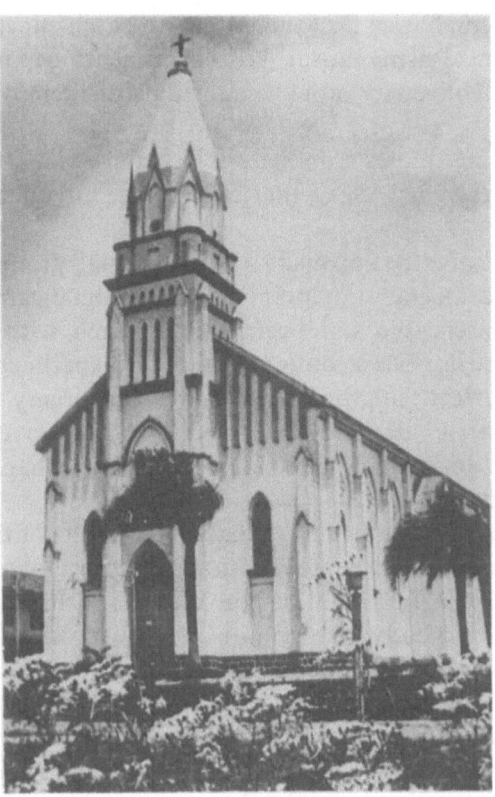

Fig. 2. Saint Stanislaw's Church.

song and dreams and uplifting clarity . . . and that the Polish motherland remains the treasurer of the national spirit and my soul, belief and language.' Nor did he ever forget, in spite of his 18 hour workdays in China, that he was a priest. 'After being at universities and doing research I have seen levels that can be reached by even electron microscopes. But I also see the unlimited borders of faith's view.'

On September 1, 1963, Father Dr Szuniewicz had a heart attack, and one month later, he had a second which required hospitalization at the Nun's Charity Hospital in Irati. On October 16, 1964, he passed away.

The above is only a brief presentation of the life of Father Dr Szuniewicz. He had many other interesting experiences, for instance the Civil War (particularly in August of 1931), the Sino-Japanese War (1937–1938), and the Chinese Civil War (1945–1949), and was always involved in missionary activities.

To bring the image of this Polish ophthalmologist closer to the readers, it is necessary to emphasize Dr Szuniewicz's research efforts on the surgical treatment of corneal astigmatism. His experiments begun in China were intensified at the University of Yale, and some of them were continued at Mafra.

The following are quotes from letters Dr Szuniewicz wrote in 1950 and 1951 from New Haven, U.S.A., that refer to the circumstances of his eye research:

'I was lucky because the university gave me a small grant of $330. It is not much but from a mortal standpoint it is very significant because it will support my research. We will begin this research with a departmental professor; it will be done as a continuation of my experiments in China. The main goal is to correct the astigmatic cornea with surgery. This project will take at least a year, so all the other projects will be delayed. I will start by using rabbits and dogs which are readily available; perhaps I will teach the critters to wear glasses!'

'Already I've buried half of my animals. The results of the latest surgical procedure to alter astigmatism are encouraging so far, but long months must pass before Dr Guida and I will be convinced that this method should be made known to everybody. We do not intend to mislead anyone and we want to be certain about the permanent results.'

'I have finished my experimental study and I am improving it in my new language. The second review of it will be done by the American physician with whom this work was done. In January the manuscript will be submitted for publication. If there is an occasion I expect to send you a reprint. I would like for Dr Rostkowski to read it.'

However, the manuscript he refers to was never submitted and thus never published. Without further explanations Dr Szuniewicz finished his experimental work at this point. However, three years later he wrote in a letter from Brazil, 'I periodically review the medical books and continue the search begun at New Haven. I have just sent in a manuscript that covers the fruits of my six long years of work, each word being carefully edited over the past two years.

If you remember, the topic of this research was my efforts to fit glasses to rabbits eyes. Lately I have been acquainted with the cats since their eye is large and they have a vertically oriented pupil that better meets my requirements. I will probably never be separated from a surgical knife ever up to my death. I am cutting and recording.'

On the basis of his correspondence we know several about the nature of his research: 1. He worked on the surgical treatment of corneal astigmatism, and to this end he performed two series of experiments. From the end of 1949 to November, 1951, he operated on some 40 rabbits and probably 9 dogs at Yale and followed them up with at least six months of observation. He then operated on an unknown number of cats at Mafra from 1952 to 1954; 2. His scientific supervisor was the ophthalmologist, Francis Paul Guida (1909–1981) – no other names appeared in his letters; 3. As a result of his work at least two manuscripts were submitted for publication, the first in January, 1952 and the second in September, 1954. For unknown reasons none of these manuscripts were published.

That is the extent of our knowledge based on the available documents about Father Dr Waclaw Szuniewicz. He started his study of the topic most likely before 1946, and certainly no later than 1948, in the Chinese town of Shuntehfu. These dates come from his letter of October 1, 1954.

Because Dr Szuniewicz's studies were never published it is likely that all this information would have been forgotten. However, his efforts have been remembered thanks to the New Haven ophthalmologist, Rocko M. Fasanella, M.D. This man knew Dr Szuniewicz, and his recollections have been added to the end of a book about him [1]. He wrote that 'Father Szuniewicz was one of the most amazing persons I ever met. He was a living saint. His medical knowledge was very modern despite being away from formal institutions for years. His laboratory studies on refractive corneal surgery from 1951 were never published, but were presented in public dissertations. These studies were independently repeated in Europe in 1976 and found to be 100% correct. He was an excellent professor in all regards.'

The book in which this appears was published in November of 1977. Four years later a paper was published in Opthalmic Surgery, entitled, 'Surgery in an Attempt to Change Corneal Curvature,' which was authored by Dr Szuniewicz and Dr Fasanella [2]. The paper presented an experimental study on 49 rabbits and dogs as well as earlier works done by other investigators prior to 1952.

Six months later another paper about refractive surgery appeared from Yale, this one being authored by Dr Fasanella alone [3]. The paper discusses various refractive surgeries, then presents a summary of Dr Szuniewicz's 1952 thesis: Surgery in an Attempt to Change Corneal Curvature; adding that he never received the information from Brazil that he had hoped for.

There are some questions which remain unanswered:
— Who received the two original manuscripts submitted by Dr Szuniewicz in December of 1952 and September of 1954, and why were they not published at that time?
— Why the manuscript, finished in 1951, was published after Dr Szuniewicz's death (1963), after Dr Guida's death (1981), and after publishing Father Stawarski's book (1977)?

In spite of minor questions such as these we feel it is evident that Father

Szuniewicz was a skilled practitioner with extensive experience in ophthalmology and a great researcher in the field of refractive surgery. The concept of the surgical correction of corneal astigmatism occurred to Dr Szuniewicz most likely before 1946 in the town of Shuntehfu, at a time when he had no access to ophthalmic literature for 21 years! We feel it is safe to say that his ideas were original and arose independently, and that his research was not simply the repeated work of others.

We have presented a hitherto unknown aspect of this great man's ophthalmologic practice and theories. It is important to realize that he equally accomplished things in the course of missionary work which would require a separate paper to outline fully.

References

1. Stawarski F. Sylwetka duchowa ksiedza doktora Waclawa Szuniewicza, Curitiba, 1977.
2. Szuniewicz W, Fasanella RM. Surgery in an attempt to change corneal curvature. Ophthalmic Surg. 1981; 12/10: 719–726.
3. Fasanella RM. Refractive Surgery. Trans. Ophthal. Soc. U.K. 1982; 102/2: 282–290.

Note: Further references may be obtained from Andrzej W. Fryczkowski. For address see below.

Address for correspondence: Dr A.W. Fryczkowski, The Ohio State University, Dept. of Ophthalmology, 456 West Tenth Avenue, Columbus, OH 93210, USA.

Documenta Ophthalmologica **74**: 57–85, 1990.
© 1990 *Kluwer Academic Publishers.*

On the history of deformation phosphenes and the idea of internal light generated in the eye for the purpose of vision

OTTO-JOACHIM GRÜSSER & MICHAEL HAGNER
Department of Physiology, Arnimallee 22, 1 Berlin 33 (West), FRG

Key words: deformation phosphenes, retina, history of ophthalmology, sensory physiology

Abstract. *Deformation phosphenes* are light sensations evoked by deformation of the eyeball in total darkness. They were first reported in Western literature by Alcmaeon of Croton in the fifth century B.C. The phenomenon of deformation phosphenes was instrumental in prompting some pre-Socratic philosophers and Plato to conceive the idea that efferent light is emitted from the eye for the purpose of vision and a '*cone of vision*' is formed by interaction with the external light. In the theories of vision this cone of vision played an important role as a signal-transmitting structure and was also used by the Greek opticians as a geometrical construction to explain optical properties of vision.

The impact of the deformation phosphene experiment on the ideas of visual sensation can be followed from Greek antiquity through the period of Roman dominance and Galen's medical teaching on to medieval times and up to the late Renaissance when, based on the anatomy of the eye as illustrated by Felix Platter, the image formation on the retina was correctly described for the first time by Johannes Kepler. In the generations following, deformation phosphenes were still employed as an important argument in defence of the theories of vision. However, the idea of physical light generated by eyeball deformation was rejected with increasing frequency during the 17th and 18th centuries. The literature on this topic is discussed, comprising the contributions of the Arabic philosophers and physicians of the 9th and 10th centuries A.D., the Franciscan and Dominican philosophers of the 13th century, Nicolaus Cusanus of the 15th century, several anatomists of the 16th and 17th centuries, Kepler, Plempius, Descartes, Boyle, Newton and others. After Kepler, the mechanical interpretation of the deformation phosphene being caused by direct action of the eyeball deformation onto the retina slowly became dominant, and the idea that physical light is generated in the eye disappeared.

The *experimentum crucis* in this matter was performed by *Giovanni Battista Morgagni* (1682–1771) and repeated and extended by *Georg August Langguth* (1711–1782). On the basis of their results, the case for physical light being generated in the eye by deformation was refuted definitively and slowly vanished thereafter from scientific literature. Deformation phosphenes were used in the 19th and 20th centuries as an instructive example of the percepts evoked by inadequate stimulation of a sense organ. J.E. Pŭrkyne in particular contributed to the study of deformation phosphenes, and finally in 1978, F. Tyler devoted a careful study to the differences between monocular and binocular deformation phosphenes. Finally some remarks on the *neurophysiological* interpretation of deformation phosphenes, based on microelectrode recordings of the activity of single retinal ganglion cells, are added to the historical report.

58

1. Introduction

When the eyeball is indented in total darkness, within less than 200 milliseconds an oval or quarter-moon shaped spot of light is perceived in the part of the visual field corresponding to the indented region of the retina. In the seconds following, this *phosphene* extends across the whole visual field and alters in structure during further eyeball indentation. It is then seen as irregular large bright spots of light, finely structured moving light grains ('light nebula') and stationary bright stars. Regular geometrical patterns appear only when both eyes are indented simultaneously [1]. When the eyeball deformation is released, part of the retina again lights up for another one or two seconds and curved light lines are seen following the course of the larger retinal vessels (Fig. 1). In the following we will review the history of this phenomenon, which played an important role during the first 2200 years of vision theories and in the development of models to explain normal vision.

2. Pre-Socratic philosophers, Plato and Aristotle

Alcmaeon of Croton (6–5th century B.C.), who was a member of the Pythagoraean sect and one of the founders of Greek medicine, was the first to describe mechanical deformation of the eyeball leading to light sensations. According to Aristotle's pupil *Theophrast of Eresos*, Alcmaeon reported that '*the eye obviously has fire within, for when the eye is struck fire flashes out*' [2, p. 88]. This observation was included in the theory of vision by another Greek physician, *Empedocles* (419–430 B.C.), who became famous for his medical and political success in the Greek colony of Akragas (Agrigente) in Sicily, but was later exiled by his countrymen. According to the fragmentary reports on Empedocles' deliberations, he also developed distinct ideas on the function of the sense organs including vision [3, p. 342; 2, p. 7–24]. He believed the eye to be composed essentially of the 'elements' *water* and *fire*. From the observations of deformation phosphenes and the lighting-up of animal eyes in the dark, he presumably deduced that internal light generated in the eye is used for the purpose of vision and that the visual percept is caused by an interaction of '*external fire*' from the objects regarded and '*internal fire*' generated by the perceiving eye [4]. This interaction takes place either somewhere within the eye or in the extrapersonal space (Fig. 2a), and follows the general rule of sensory perception postulated by Empedocles and some of the other pre-Socratic philosophers, that perception is only possible when the physiological process in the sense organ is similar to the

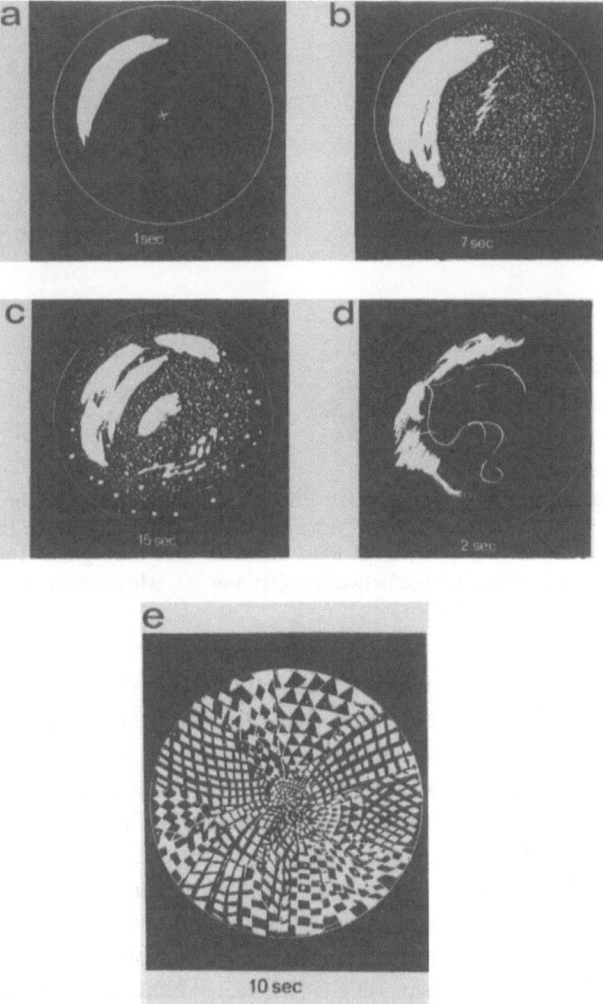

Fig. 1. Development of deformation phosphenes after indentation of the temporal side of the right eyeball at different intervals following indentation (a–c) and after release of eyeball deformation (d), as seen by one of the authors (O.-J. G.). (e) With simultaneous bilateral indentation of both eyeballs on the temporal side of the eye a patterned deformation phosphene is observed, flickering at about 10 Hz. The figure (e) represents the impression after about 10 seconds of indentation.

physical signal in the outer world. Other Greek natural philosophers postulated just the opposite and assumed that perception occurs by *contrast* between signal and sensory process [2].

A generation after Empedocles, *Democritus of Abdera* (460–370 B.C.),

60

Empedokles (-490 – 430 v.Chr.)

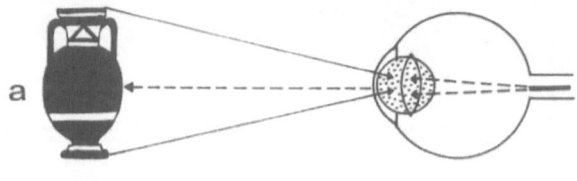

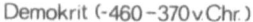

Demokrit (-460 –370 v.Chr.)

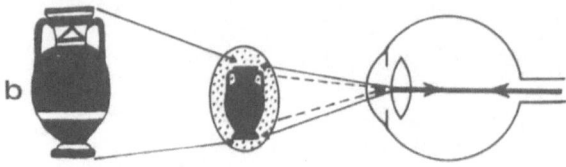

Fig. 2. (a) Interaction-theory of Empedocles: Efferent light is generated in the eye, leaves it, touches the object and is reflected back to the eye for the purpose of vision. (b) Democritus modified this interaction theory: Efferent light interacts with the signals from the objects somewhere in the extrapersonal space between object and eye, where small impressions of the object are generated in the air [74].

who together with his teacher *Leukippos* founded Greek materialistic philosophy, developed more explicit thoughts on the interaction of efferent and afferent visual signal flow. He believed that the process of visual perception uses small impressions, called in Greek *'typoi'*, which are generated in the air by fine material images (*'ediola'*) composed of atoms, travelling from the objects towards the eye and interacting with internal light evoked in and leaving the eye of the perceiving subject (Fig. 2b). Thus, Democritus assumed that perception occurs only when an extrapersonal interaction of efferent and afferent light has taken place [2].

Although *Plato* (Athens, 427–347 B.C.) disliked the materialistic philosophy of Democritus, he seriously considered models of vision along the same lines and developed a more specific theory of vision (Fig. 3) in his most important book on natural philosophy, *'Timaeus'* [5, 45b–d]. He assumed that 'visual rays' are emitted from the eye and form by interaction with the external light a signal-transmitting structure, the *'body of vision'* or *'cone of vision'*, as it was later called by *Euclid* and *Ptolemy* [6]. This body of vision was believed to touch the objects and to be moved by this interaction. The movement is reflected back to the eye, which receives and transmits it to the brain, inducing mechanisms of visual cognition. In this model of vision, which was later called *'synaugia'*, perception by touch became the dominant principle in the models for sensory perception.

Platon (428 – 348 v. Chr.)

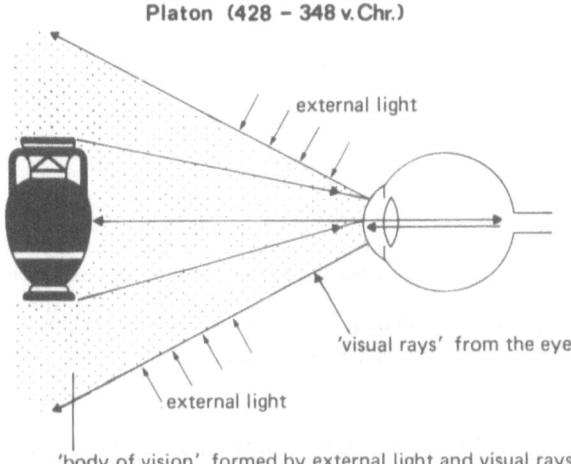

external light

'visual rays' from the eye

external light

'body of vision' formed by external light and visual rays

Fig. 3. Plato's interaction theory: Efferent visual rays are emitted from the eye and interact with the external light to form the 'body of vision'. This body of vision touches the objects. The results of this interaction are reflected back to the eye [74].

Several generations later, *Chrysippos* (277–204 B.C.), one of the leading philosophers of the early Stoa [7], on the basis of Plato's theory, proposed the existence of a spatially organized visual cone, having its base at the objects, its pinnacle in the eye [8, 9]. Chrysippos assumed that perception is always dependent on active movement directed towards the objects. Only such an intentionally controlled movement releases '*pneuma*' from the sense organs. The idea of a visual cone composed of internal light (*visual pneuma*, later called in Latin '*Spiritus visibilis*') dominated the theories of vision during Greek and Roman antiquity from the time of Plato to that of *Galen* (129–199 A.D.). *Aristotle* (384–322 B.C.) and his pupil *Theophrastus of Eresos* (372–287 B.C.) were not particularly impressed by the interaction theory and believed that vision, as perception in general, is mainly a passive process. In '*De sensu et sensato*' Aristotle rejected the idea of physical light generated within the eye and leaving the eye for the purpose of vision. He was familiar with the phenomenon of deformation phosphenes, but explained them as 'self-reflection' within the eye, caused by its '*smoothness and its natural illuminating power*', which could be evoked by eyeball deformation in complete darkness [4, 437a–b]. From the accounts of soldiers, Aristotle also knew that injury to the eye produced the impression of a burning lamp being blown out, followed by darkness [4, 438b]. This description leaves open the possibility that Aristotle recognized that an eyeball injury leads to a short transient increase in light sensation before the 'darkness', just as an oil flame, when blown out, flares up before disappearing.

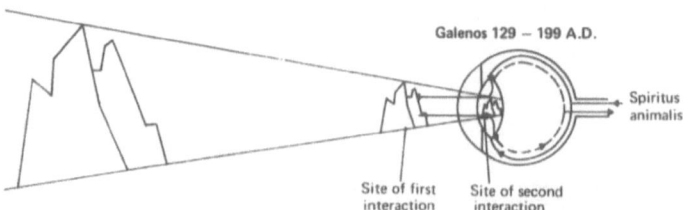

Fig. 4. The eclectic modification of the interaction theory by Galen [75]: The spiritus animalis (pneuma) generated in the brain reaches the eye and leaves it again, altering the air in front of the eye. By this mechanism the image of the object is diminished (first interaction). This reduced image reaches the crystalline body (lens), which is sensitized by the pneuma. There a second interaction occurs, which is then transmitted back to the optic nerve and from there to the brain [13].

A position similar to that of Aristotle was taken by the *Epicureans*. In his *'Letter to Herodotus'* [10] the founder of this Athenean school of philosophy, *Epicurus* (341–270 B.C.), wrote that perception is a passive process in its initial stage, followed by an active recognition mechanism (*'prolepsis'*), which depends on the subject's experience, but operates only *within the organism* and not outside of it. Thus the Epicureans rejected the idea of efferent pneuma leaving the eye for the purpose of vision.

As mentioned above, the idea of Plato's *'synaugia'* was accepted by the great Greek mathematician *Euclid* (end of 3rd century B.C.) and the astronomer *Claudius Ptolemy* (2nd century A.D.), but from their reports it is not clear whether they thought that the efferent pneuma represented more than just a geometrical construction of the *'cone of vision'* [6]. The ancient theories of vision, excluding those of the classical theory of optics, were summarized and discussed by *Galen*, who thought that the illuminating pneuma originates in the brain and reaches the eye via the optic nerves. In *'De usu partium corporis'* he supported an interaction theory similar to that proposed by Plato and Chrysippos. On the other hand, true to his eclectic approach to science, Galen also conceded that vision is possible when only the objects seen emit light directly to the eyes [11, 12, 13] (Fig. 4).

3. Medieval and Renaissance variations on the idea that light is generated in the eye

The Greek concept of efferent and afferent light interaction as a primary source in visual perception was still under discussion in medieval and Renaissance theories of vision [14]. In the early Middle Ages the Arabian physicians and scientists *Hunain Ibn Ishaq* (808–873 A.D.) and *Al-Kindi* (813–873 A.D.) supported the extrapersonal interaction theory but believed

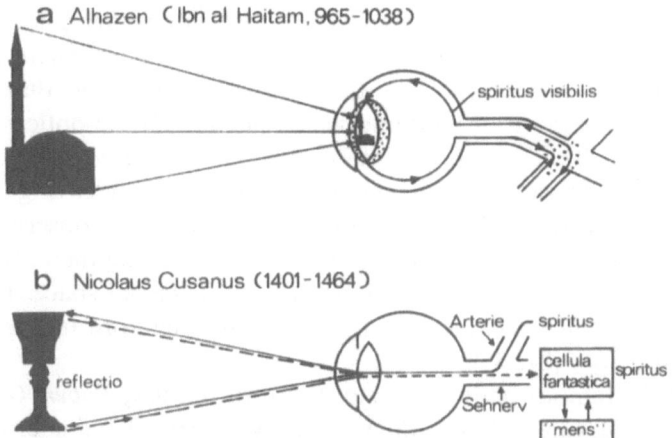

Fig. 5. (a) Alhazen's modification of the interaction theory: Efferent signals, the spiritus visibilis generated in the brain, reach the eye via the optic nerve and interact for the purpose of vision with the images of the objects formed on the crystalline lens at the site of the pupil. The modified spiritus visibilis is then sent back to the optic chiasm and from there to the brain. (b) Nikolaus Cusanus modified the old external interaction theory: The spiritus visibilis leaves the eye only when attention is cast upon certain objects. After interaction with the object, it is reflected back to the eye and transmitted via the optic nerve to the cellula phantastica, where the material spiritus visibilis interacts with the immaterial soul ('*mens*') [74].

that the emission of internal light is strictly dependent on eye movements [15, 16]. In the next generation of Arab scientists, however, *Ibn-al-Haytham* (in Latin *Alhazen*, 965–1040 A.D.) rejected the external interaction theory [17]. He developed some new ideas based on the *Optics* of *Ptolemy* and the anatomy of the eye as described by *Galen* [18, 19]. From the Latin translation of Alhazen's main book on optics, one could infer that he believed the interaction between efferent pneuma and the visual rays from the outside world to take place in the crystalline lens of the eye. He assumed that the *spiritus visibilis* is produced in the brain near the chiasm of the optic nerves and flows in small vessels through the optic nerve to the retina and within the retina to the crystalline lens, where it interacts with the object images formed there by the light of the outside world. Subsequently, the *spiritus visibilis* flows back to the optic nerve and through its channels to the chiasm, where it mixes with the afferent *spiritus visibilis* of the other eye (Fig. 5a). Alhazen was convinced of the necessity of this mechanism for correct binocular fusion. Like Aristotle, he discarded the idea that internal light leaves the eye. He also argued that efferent light inevitably would disturb the process of seeing. Recently G.A. Russell [20] studied the Arabic manuscript of Alhazen's Optics, '*Kitab al-Manazir*' and provided convincing evidence that Alhazen believed light to be refracted twice within the optics of the eye and an image formed at the *'funnel of the optic nerve'*, from where the signal is transmitted to the brain. This leads to the supposition that Alhazen assumed an interaction of light and visual pneuma in the optic nerve.

Alhazen's position was supported by *Avicenna* (*Ibn Sina* 980–1037 A.D.) who put forward a simple argument against internal light leaving the eye. If this theory were correct, he wrote, the presence of many observers would improve the perception properties of the air surrounding them, since more visual pneuma would be released into the extrapersonal space. Evidently, this could be refuted empirically and Avicenna therefore rejected Plato's interaction theory [21, 22].

Among the famous philosophers of the 13th century, *Robert Grosseteste* (ca. 1168–1253), Chancellor of the University of Oxford and later Bishop of Lincoln, supported the idea of internal light leaving the eye for the purpose of vision. Grosseteste wrote: *'One should not assume that the emission of rays from the eye is only apparent and without reality. This is the opinion of those, who know parts, but do not consider the whole. One should understand that the visual species emitted from the eye is a substance which illuminates similarly as the sun. These emitted rays complete the act of vision when they join those from the objects of the extrapersonal space'* [23, p. 72–73]. He considered light to be the elementary substance of the world and consequently to have a metaphysical function far beyond vision.

The most important follower of Robert Grosseteste within the next generation of Oxford Franciscans was *Roger Bacon* (1214–1292). He was not only interested in scientific experimentation but was also well-read in Greek and Arabic medical texts. He rejected Alhazen's model of vision, the concept of higher activity with a physiological mechanism inside the eye, but emphasized the Platonic teaching of pneuma and that a special vital 'species' i.e., a signal, is emitted by the eyes and reaches the objects of vision [24]. He believed that *'The species of the things of the world are not suited to act immediately and fully on sight because of the nobility of the latter. Therefore these species must be aided and excited by the species of the eye, which proceeds through the locale of the visual pyramid, altering and ennobling the medium and rendering it commensurate with sight; and thus it prepares for the approach of the species of the visible object [itself], so that it is altogether conformable and commensurate with the nobility of the animated body, i.e., the eye.'* [24, p. 52].

Albertus Magnus (1197–1280), the great teacher of the Dominican order, also reported that light is seen during eyeball deformation, but rejected the idea of light leaving the eye. This was not the only scientific dissent regarding the function of sense organs between the English Franciscans and the continental Dominicans of that time. Albert wrote: '. . . *A certain sensation appears in the eyes in darkness, either when they are compressed from outside or suddenly beaten: then a lightening fire is generated in the eye and it would not light up inside if it would not be inside'* (25, Quaestio XX, ad. 11). As a possible interpretation of the deformation phosphenes Albert discussed: *'. . . that the cause is the transluminance* [claritas] *of the spiritus visibilis, which extends in itself by the bending or beating* [of the eye]. *Therefore a luminous variation appears in the rear of the eye . . .'* [25, Quaestio, XX, ad. 11].

Albert conjectured furthermore that the *spiritus visibilis* interacts with the form of the visual images *inside the eye*, most probably at the site of the crystalline lens (Fig. 5a). Only in the case of some nocturnal animals, such as cats and wolves, did he still believe that light is generated inside the eye and might leave it for the purpose of vision [25, Quaestio XIX].

The Parisian *Jean Buridan* (1295–1358), one of the leading nominalistic and aristotelian philosophers of his time, while commenting on Aristotle's book in his *'Quaestiones super librum de sensu et sensato'*, mentioned that the appearance of phosphenes does not support the idea of efferent light and the Platonic interaction theory. He argued, as Alhazen, that light generated in the eye would be permanently visible for the observer and would therefore interfere with normal vision. Buridan wrote on deformation phosphenes: *'. . . but when the eye is struck it* [the light] *is bent inward and thus one part reflects light into another part* [of the eye] *and vice versa; therefore one part perceives 'lux' through 'lumen' reflected by the other part'* [14, p. 135].

Despite the strong arguments against emission of internal light, this hypothesis still had supporters during the 15th century. *Nicolaus Cusanus* (1401–1464), for example, a philosopher, mathematician and church politician of great repute, presented a variant of the old interaction theory in his books *'Compendium'* [26] and *'Liber de mente'* and a generalization thereof for the other senses: *'Because the spiritus is an instrument of the senses, the eyes, the nose and the other sense organs can be considered to be windows through which the spiritus has its exit for the purpose of perception'* [27, p. 257].

Cusanus believed that two arteries transport a highly movable type of *spiritus visibilis* to the eye, which then leaves the eye and hits the objects in the extrapersonal space. Thereafter the spiritus visibilis is reflected back to the eye and, after some refinement, reaches the *cellula phantastica* of the brain via the optic nerve. *Cellula phantastica* was the name for the lateral ventricles of the brain, the place where Cusanus believed the immaterial soul *'mens'* to be aroused by an exchange of information (*phantasma*) with the very fine, but material *spiritus visibilis* from the eye. The result of this exchange is transmitted to the third cerebral ventricle in the middle part of the brain, the *cellula rationis*, thought to be the seat of the immaterial, rational argumentation and insight. In accordance with ancient Stoic teaching, Cusanus supported the idea that the generation of *spiritus visibilis* has something to do with motor acts, i.e., the emission of the spiritus visibilis depends on *spatially selective attention* being directed towards the object one wishes to see (Fig. 5b).

4. Further modifications of Alcmaeon's and Plato's hypothesis on deformation phosphenes and the development of a new theory of vision based on Renaissance anatomy

Towards the second half of the 16th and the first half of the 17th centuries, the field of anatomy advanced considerably and the body of information on the structure of the sense organs gained in empirical foundation. Improved knowledge of eye structures also led to gradual changes in their functional interpretation. The anatomist *Girolamo (Hieronymus) Fabricius ab Aquapendente* (1537–1619), who taught at the University of Padova, gave a fairly correct description of the anatomy of the eye in his tractate '*De actione oculorum*' and rejected the idea of light emitted from the eye. He took the cone of vision only as a *geometrical construction* to explain why vision with one eye is restricted to a certain part of the extrapersonal space. He considered the retina to be the light-sensitive structure, but finally opted for the old dogma that the crystalline lens is where the image is transformed into a physiological process [28, p. 203ff; 29].

The great clinician and anatomist from the University of Basel, *Felix Platter (Plater,* 1536–1614), deeply impressed by the 'new anatomy' of *Andreas Vesalius*, described the anatomy of the eye somewhat more realistically than Fabricius, depicted the lens in its proper position and drew the curvature of its surfaces correctly [30, 31]. Platter's anatomy of the eye was adapted by *Caspar Bauhin* (1560–1624), who in 1589 became professor of anatomy at the University of Basel, but in Bauhin's books '*De corporis humani fabrica, libri IV*' [32] and '*Theatrum anatomicum*' [33, p. 706ff, Tab XIX] the Galenic tradition, that the crystal lens is the sensitive organ for vision, was still supported. The older Felix Platter, however, was more progressive and attributed this function to the retina, but he still did not understand the image formation on the retina correctly.

Based on the anatomical findings and speculations of Platter, the famous Suebian astronomer *Johannes Kepler* (1571–1630) was finally able to reject the age-old concept that the transductive mechanisms between external light and physiological processes are located in the crystal lens of the eye. In his book '*Paralipomena ad Vittelonem. . .*' in 1604 Kepler, applying the laws of refraction by optical surfaces, proposed that an *inverted image* of the object is cast onto the inner surface of the retina and assumed that this structure is also responsible for the transduction of external light into a physiological process, which is then transmitted by the optic nerve to the brain [34, 35]. Kepler also deliberated over a new explanation for deformation phosphenes. He maintained that the *mechanical irritation of the iris* by eyeball deformation induces sparks which stimulate the retina. Thus, he still believed that 'physical' light is generated in the eye during the perception of deformation phosphenes, but as the source of this light he selected a structure in the eye not directly involved in the process of vision. His arguments for light generation in the iris by eyeball deformation were rather indirect: '*the light can impossibly have its seat in the moistures of the eye* [i.e., crystal lens and vitreous body], *because then it would disturb the process of vision*' [35, 36, 37].

Kepler's contemporary, the Jesuit Father *Christoph Scheiner* (1579–1650), followed the idea that during the perception of deformation phosphenes physical light is generated in the eye, but he believed it to be produced in the crystal lens and normally too weak to be seen. Only when the mechanical stimulation releases a large amount of this internal light, as in the case of deformation phosphenes, can it be seen. Scheiner performed several important experiments in visual psychophysics and also gave a detailed description of deformation phosphenes, observing the correlation between the position of the phosphene in the visual field and the site of the retina indented: '*The appearance* [of the phosphene] *is round. But if the pressure is stronger the perceived light extends and finally takes an elliptic form. One always perceives it on the opposite side* [in the visual field] *to where the eye is deformed. The spark is mainly to be seen in the darkness, independent of whether the eyelids are closed or open. But one perceives it even by day and with open eyes, especially near the angle of eye. The whole appearance consists of a gleaming border, it is then in the middle dark and nearly black*' [38, p. 238].

Accordingly, Scheiner contributed three new ideas to the traditional description of deformation phosphenes:

a) deformation phosphenes depend on the amount of pressure exerted onto the eye;
b) phosphenes evoked in darkness differ from those seen in light;
c) the initial phosphene is perceived opposite the site of deformation, an observation corroborating Kepler's concept of functional reversion of the retina.

Scheiner believed that the internal light illuminates the crystal lens and this illumination is reflected to and perceived by the retina. Like Kepler, he assumed that the phosphenes are a kind of *real light* and are caused by mechanical processes within the eye. In the opinion of both, however, intraocular light was a curiosity rather than anything of great importance to the process of normal vision.

Kepler's description of image formation in the eye only gained slow acceptance among the anatomists of his time, despite the fact that he based his theory on the anatomical figures of Felix Platter and had collaborated with the anatomist *Johannes Jessen* (1566–1621) of Prague during his years as Habsburg court astronomer and astrologer of *Wallenstein*. In 1632, for example, the Dutch anatomist and physician *Plempius* (Plemp) published a book '*Ophthalmographia*', in which he mentioned Kepler's '*Dioptrice*' but was hesitant to introduce the '*teaching of the mathematicians*' into medicine. He attributed the idea of the retina being the organ of light sensation to Fabricius ab Aquapendente [39], but most likely did not understand the constructions of the dioptrics of the eye published a quarter of a century before by Johannes Kepler. *Vopiscus Fortunatus Plempius* (1601–1671) is known to posterity as a correspondence partner of Descartes on the matter of perception and on Harvey's concept of blood circulation. He was trained in Leyden, Padova and Bologna and taught from 1633 as professor at the Faculty of Medicine at Loewen. Plempius was a convinced Aristotelian, opposed heavily to the spread of Cartesian ideas at the university [40]. In his '*Ophthalmographia*' he devoted a full chapter to phosphenes. Under the heading '*What is the cause for our incidental perception of flashes or moving sparks in the eyes?*' he described phosphenes visible when the eye is pressed or rubbed [39, p. 237–240]. He also mentioned phosphenes seen during fast saccadic eye movements in the dark and was well acquainted with the traditional ideas on phosphene generation. He rejected Scheiner's hypothesis that physical light is generated inside the eye and assumed that the light sensations caused by eyeball deformation are evoked by a change in the flow of the spiritus visibilis in the eye: Due to the mechanically increased speed of the spiritus the latter is 'inflamed'. He believed that the same phenomenon also occurred by a chemical process caused by additional gases ('*vapores*') mixed to the spiritus by the mechanical forces during eyeball deformation. Thus Plempius favoured a mechano-chemical hypothesis of phosphene generation. He emphasized that this internal '*ignition*' is relatively mild. Therefore phosphenes are not seen when the deformed eye looks simultaneously at a bright external light, which is then believed to mask the '*glare of the spiritus*' in a similar manner as the light of the sun masks the light of the stars during the daytime.

Kepler's idea on the dioptrics of the eye and vision in general undoubtedly had some impact on *René Descartes* (1596–1650). In his books '*Dioptrique*' [41] and '*Tractatus de homine*' [42] Descartes accepted Kepler's construction of the inverted retinal image. He believed that light acting on the retina exerts a direct mechanical influence on the optic nerve, being transmitted according to the laws of mechanics by means of small fibers located inside the tubular nerve channels to the central projection regions of the optic nerve. As *Leonardo da Vinci* (1452–1519) a century before [43, Codex D, folio 5 recto], he assumed the latter to be located along the walls of the lateral ventricles of the brain and explained the deformation phosphenes according to this mechanical model:

'. . . *remember those whose eyes will be beaten. They believed to see light flashes, although their eyelids are closed or they are in a dark room. Therefore the origin of this sensation can only be the power or the blow on the eye, which moves the small fibers of the optic nerves equally as light does*' [41, p. 31].

With these remarks Descartes clearly rejected, as Plempius at that time, the idea that *physical light* was generated within the eye. A similar position was taken by the English chemist *Robert Boyle* (1627–1691), who described deformation phosphenes in his book '*Experiments and considerations touching colours*' [44]. He also believed that external light acts on the retina by means of mechanical interaction:

'*But I will rather observe that not only when a man receives a great stroke upon his eye or a very great one upon some other part of his head, he is wont to see, as it were, flashes of lightning, and little vivid, but vanishing flames, though perhaps his eyes be shut; but the like apparitions may happen, when the motion proceeds not from something without, but from something within the body, provided the unwanted fumes that wander up and down in the head, or the propagated concussion of any internal part in the body, to cause about the inward extremities of the optic nerve, such a motion as is wont to be there produced, when the stroke of the light upon the retina makes us conclude, that we see either light or such and such a colour*' [44, p. 671–672].

It is not clear what Boyle meant precisely by '*fumes*', but it is evident that he followed, in general, the mechanistic concepts of Plempius and Descartes and did not support the old hypothesis of physical light evoked by mechanical eyeball irritation. As another example of visual sensations evoked by mechanical irritation of the eye, Boyle mentioned phosphenes seen during a fit of coughing.

Similarly, the Cartesians of the generation following Descartes usually explained the deformation phosphenes by mechanical irritation of the retina. *Johannes Clauberg* (1622–1665), for example, who was the most active promotor of Cartesian thought in Germany and as professor of philosophy taught at the University of Duisburg during the last decade of his life (45), assumed that the light perceived on mechanical irritation or injury of the eye is caused by a mechanical activation of the *spiritus visibilis* inside the retina, which is then transmitted into the brain. There, he believed, the essential mechanisms of perception occur. Since Clauberg was a strict *occasionalist* who postulated *psychophysical parallelism* without any causal connections between body and soul ('*mens*'), he believed that the unusual activation of spiritus visibilis by eyeball deformation is automatically paralleled by a corresponding light sensation of the immaterial soul. He compared the activation of the spiritus visibilis in the eye by mechanical irritation with the similar 'turbulence' of the spiritus occurring inside the brain during the state of vertigo [46, p. 196].

The French Cartesian *Nicolas Malebranche* (1638–1715) discussed deformation phosphenes, applying a strict occasionalistic interpretation: '*Due to the pressure exerted onto the eye, one perceives light, despite no illuminated body being present. This is caused by the pressure exerted by the finger onto the eye and therefore also onto the brain . . . The light one perceives, is a property of mental activity and as a consequence is only found in this sphere. . .*' [47, p. 94–95]. Malebranche pointed out that the light is not seen at the site where the eyeball is indented, but in the extrapersonal space opposite. He explained this by the assumption that '*the pressure of the finger on the left* [indented] *side of the eyeball has the same effect as an illuminated body seen on the right side . . .*' [47, p. 95]. Malebranche applied Kepler's idea of the inverted retinal image to explain the localisation of the deformation phosphenes, whereby his arguments were deduced from the '*divine laws*', '*which were arranged by God to save in his design (of the organism) complete unity*' [47, p. 95].

Thomas Bartholinus (1616–1680), professor of anatomy at the University of Copenhagen, wrote a comprehensive monograph on the importance of light in men and animals [48]. He discussed extensively older reports on light believed to be emitted from the eyes of men, especially those of great political repute, such as the Roman emperors *Augustus* or *Tiberius*, and described meticulously ways of eliciting deformation phosphenes: '*It is true without doubt that when the eyes are pressed near the angle of the orbit that even in total darkness, whenever the indenting finger moves, a real light lights up. It disappears when the eyelids are moved away and reappears when the eyelids are pressed* [towards the eyeball]. *I can confirm from my own experience that everybody can perceive this light in his eyes when he follows this procedure. It is certain that by slight compression* [of the eyes] *only mild light is evoked. Yet the stronger one presses, the stronger the fist is moved to the eyes, the stronger light scintillations appear, in the same manner as sparks are evoked when flintstones are struck against each other. . .'* [48, p. 109]. Bartholinus, however, still believed that some animal eyes, like those of cats, can emit real light in the dark for the purpose of vision [48, p. 249–250].

In the second half of the 17th century in his book '*Ophthalmographia*' [49] the English physician and ophthalmologist *William Briggs* (1642–1704) continued to defend the old idea of 'real' internal light generated in the eyeball by deformation. He believed that the *spiritus visibilis* acts within the retina, begins to gleam when the eyeball is deformed and stimulates the retina in a way similar to natural light projected from the oustide world. With this hypothesis Briggs contradicted Kepler and Scheiner, as he could not understand how a liquid structure such as the lens could generate light when pressure acted on it.

Towards the end of the 17th century the mechanical model of deformation phosphenes became clearly dominant. *Isaac Newton* (1643–1727) also rejected the idea that physical light is generated by eyeball deformation. In book 3, part I of his '*Opticks*' he wrote in *Quaerie* 16:

'*When a man in the dark presses either corner of his eye with his finger, and turns his eye away from his finger, he will see a circle of colours like those in the feather of a peacock's tail. If the eye and the finger remain quiet these colours vanish in a second minute of time, but if the finger be moved with a quavering motion they appear again. Do not these colours arise from such motions, excited in the bottom of the eye by the pressure and motion of the finger, as, at other times are excited there by light for causing vision? And do not these motions once excited continue about a second of time before they cease? And when a man by a stroke upon his eyes sees a flash of light, are not the like motions excited in the retina by the stroke? . . . And considering the lastingness of the motions excited in the bottom of the eye by light, are they not of a vibrating nature?*' [50, p. 347].

Accordingly Newton's explanation of deformation phosphenes avoided the hypothesis of gleaming animal spirits. He preferred to defend the direct transduction from mechanical vibration of the retina into sensation rather than to follow Brigg's speculations.

5. The experimental refutation of the idea that physical light is generated in the deformed eye

It is evident that with Kepler's concept of the inverted image which is transformed in the retina into a physiological process, a theory of vision no longer required the hypothesis of light generated in the eye. Nevertheless, the deformation phosphenes remained an interesting phenomenon for those discussing the elementary mechanisms of vision. The phosphene was still interpreted as a kind of 'activated' internal light and thus became a link between new theories of vision in the 17th century and the traditional interpretations. The reason for this was the limited use of Kepler's theory of vision by himself, by Scheiner and by Briggs. A consistent application of Kepler's image formation theory was performed by Descartes and his successors and by Newton. Their concept of a mechanical process underlying all sensation, applied to the theory of vision, became a plausible explanation for the phosphene, replacing the older theories.

The final *experimental* refutation of the age-old postulate that physical light is generated in the eye by eyeball deformation or blows to the eyeball did not come about until the beginning of the 18th century. It was *Giovanni Battista Morgagni* (1682–1771), one of the leading Italian anatomists of his time, who furnished the experimental evidence to directly reject the generation of physical light within the deformed eye. In his '*Adversaria anatomica omnia*' [51] he devoted one chapter to ophthalmology in which he also discussed the deformation phosphenes. He sided with William Briggs against Christoph Scheiner and pointed out that pressure exerted on the cornea and transmitted directly to the crystal lens could not be the cause of any light sensation. Similarly, he opposed Kepler's view that the iris could generate light. Morgagni also observed that deformation of the eyeball on two sides leads to two phosphenes:

> As I observed repeatedly it is certain that no light appears when the cornea is pressed. When, however, the region near the cornea is deformed, light appears immediately in the shape of half an annulus. Deformation a little further away produces a light annulus. If during the same time two regions of the eyeball are deformed, two light rings appear immediately. When, however, the pressure is exerted not only with the finger tips but with the whole finger, the light takes on an elliptic form. Applying instead of the finger a much smaller round body, such as the head of a needle, the light ring is much smaller. It always appears on the side [of the visual field] opposite that indented' [51, p. 92].

Morgagni believed that the phosphenes are caused by '*stretch of the fibers of the tunica retiformis'* [i.e., the retina] and assumed that by these *'vibrations, the animal spirit is affected as it is by the rays of light.'* Finally with the help of an assistant he performed a simple and elegant experiment in a dark room, demonstrating that no light is generated by mechanical irritation of the eyeball. When Morgagni deformed his eye with his finger and perceived bright phosphenes, the other person was asked to see whether light leaves Morgagni's eye, but *'even when he observed extremely carefully and very bright light appeared to me* [Morgagni], *he could never observe any light by himself'* [51, p. 93]. From the outcome of this expeirment and his previous experimental observations, Morgagni concluded that deformation in excised eyes did not produce any light and that the phosphenes are entirely *subjective.* As an explanation for their existence he assumed a *mechanical irritation of the spiritus visibilis.* Morgagni performed his deformation phosphene experiments not only out of theoretical interest but also with practical goals in mind. He believed that the apparition of the light cycle caused by eyeball deformation in the dark can be taken as an indication of normal retinal function. Thus he argued that a pressure phosphene seen by patients suffering from cataract of the lens is a positive prognostic criterion for the ophthalmic surgeon: when he removes the opaque crystal lens, the patient's chances of regaining his vision are fairly good [51, p. 94].

Morgagni's publication came into the hands of *Georg August Langguth* (1711–1782), a German physician working at that time at the famous *University of Wittenberg.* He had taught anatomy and botany there since 1742 and held a chair in both since 1747. His bibliography contains nearly 70 papers, dealing mainly with surgical topics. His dissertation *'De luce ex pressione oculi'* [52] was published in 1742 when he became a member of the medical faculty.* This paper seems to be Langguth's only contribution to sensory physiology.

In the introduction to his essay, Langguth wrote that he perceived the phosphene for the first time by chance, but before setting up his experiments, he was evidently also acquainted with Morgagni's description of the phosphenes in *'Adversaria anatomica omnia'.* Langguth performed his experiments in an absolutely dark room and deformed his eyeball with a finger or an ivory ball the size of a pea mounted on a small stick. He described how the phosphene *'always appears opposite the deformation site'* [52, p. IV]. To find out whether physical light is generated in the eyeball by the deformation, he observed his deformed eye in a mirror in the dark and tried to see whether in addition to the phosphene he could discover light appearing at

---

* One copy of Langguths *'De luce ex pressione oculi'* is extant at the Herzog August Bibliothek, Wolfenbüttel.

the spot where he believed he should see his pupil. Finally he repeated Morgagni's experiment:

'*A friend, who became curious about these phenomena . . . visited me in the dark room. I briefly explained to him what I was doing. The doors were closed and I asked him to observe my eyes very closely. While I was perceiving the small lights* [i.e., the deformation phosphenes] *he was not able to observe any small flashes or oscillating lights. Thereafter he performed the same experiment by himself according to the same rules, experimental procedure and design. He was asked to confirm whether light appears to him immediately by pressure on the eye. I, however, could not discover any light leaving his eyes. Later I performed this experiment repeatedly, always with the same result; in the middle of the night or when I was lying horizontally, early in the morning when I awoke from sleep before sunrise. Even when I covered one eye for the whole day and occluded* [during the experiment] *the other eye with the hand, the described pressure on the eye led to the same effect. Similarly, when I opened one eye, observed the normally illuminated objects, closed the other eye and pressed on it, the same light sensations appeared, but somewhat weaker*' [52, p. VI].*

Langguth explained his observations by a rather traditional model of vision: the image of the object affects the retina and alters immediately the spiritus animalis. This alteration is transmitted to the brain by the spiritus flow and activates the immaterial mind within the brain, which directs its attention to the object. The action of the spiritus animalis in the retina is governed by certain chemical processes. He applied the same idea to explain the appearance of the deformation phosphenes:

'*The particles at hand* [of the animal spirit] *are gathered together and somehow mingled with the liquid, oily, most subtle fluids. The eyelid is held very slightly away from the eyeball by mechanical pressure, when the eyelids are firmly closed and a vacuum is generated. This causes the flash of light to appear*' [52, p. XIII].

Langguth's physico-chemical hypothesis of the deformation phosphenes is not very clear. Apparently he thought that mechanical pressure would lead to an *interaction of the retina and the vitreous body* at their contiguous surfaces. This would change some properties of the vitreous body, which are transmitted to the *spiritus animalis* in the retina.

* German translation of Langguth's '*dissertatio*' in Hagner 1987, p. 132–142.

Morgagni's and Langguth's observations and explanations could be considered a modification of Plempius' and Decartes' mechanical theory on pressure phosphenes, although both did not mention either of them. Langguth only referred to those authors whose names he had read in Morgagni's book. Somewhat unjustly he criticized the theory of Kepler, Scheiner and Briggs, mentioned above, and was convinced that their explanations of the pressure phosphenes had not advanced the comprehension of this phenomenon [52, p. XIV]. On the other hand, he developed a stringent mechano-chemical theory, whereby he was aware of the fact that his theoretical assumptions were rather speculative.

In a quite amicable manner Morgagni mentioned Langguth's experiments in his major opus 'De sedibus et causis morborum' [53, 54]:

'My profound wish was to read the thoughts of the most admirable Mr. Georg August Langguth. In his dissertation on the light apparition, he not only affirmed my statements but also confirmed them with his own experiments. Accordingly, when one would explain in particular and not in general that which we both observed in the same question and especially that which he performed with a friend, one would easily recognize which of the two premises are most suitable' [54, p. 598].

Comparing Langguth's and Morgagni's studies on the deformation phosphenes, one empirical step forward has been made in the report of the former: He refers to the fact that in principle, pressure phosphenes do not change during the course of dark adaptation. We repeated these dark adaptation experiments and could confirm Langguth's observation: The pressure phosphenes appear to be about the same, whether in a photopic-adapted retina within the first minute after the light is turned off or under scotopic adaptation conditions after the subject has remained for one hour in a totally dark room [55].

6. The discussion of deformation phosphenes in the physiological literature of the 18th, 19th and early 20th centuries

Morgagni's and Langguth's explanation of the deformation phosphenes and their rejection of the idea of physical light generated in the eye were accepted by the physiologists of following generations. Soon their names no longer appeared in the textbooks, only their experiments and results. *Herman Boerhaave* (1668–1738), the eminent clinician from the University of Leyden, mentioned the deformation phosphenes in his textbooks on vision and the disease of the eye [56]. He described phosphenes on different occasions, attributed them to mechanical irritation of the optic nerve, and observed light sensations not only when the eye was directly indented but also affected by other mechanical forces: '*Whenever we sneeze in darkness or cough, we can perceive light sparks, and the same is true when someone hits against our head or the eye . . . This is no real light but only a change in the shape of the eye together with the compression of the optic nerve or the retina, and these changes produce the same sensation of light, which normally are evoked by the refracted light beams. Whenever the optic nerve is moved as it is moved by the light, independent of which cause moves it, the same impression of light is evoked . . .*' [56, p. 121]. Boerhaave mentioned that when infections or other diseases affect the eye, light sensations are particularly easy to evoke by pressure on the eye in total darkness. He considered this phenomenon as a bad sign for the prognosis of the disease, indicating the danger of total blindness. Boerhaave rejected the traditional idea that cats, horses or other animals emit light from their eyes in the dark for the purpose of vision. It was evident to him that in total darkness the only advantage these animals had over man was that their pupils could dilate more so that the retina could catch more light from the surroundings [56, p. 193].

Boerhaaves pupil, the Swiss-born *Albrecht von Haller* (1708–1777), professor of anatomy and physiology at the University of Göttingen, who became famous in the neurosciences because of his intensive discussion on the sensibility (*sensibilitas*) of the nerve and the irritability (*irritabilitas*) of the muscles, devoted a small chapter of his eight-volume Physiology Handbook to the phosphenes [57]. He followed Boerhaave in emphasizing the effect of mechanical pressure exerted on the retina by eyeball deformation and conjectured that physical light also causes mechanical pressure on the retina. Therefore the same percept, namely light is evoked: '*It is . . . a useful dogma that our soul cannot discriminate equal percepts and attributes the* [perceptual] *consequences of an unknown cause to another, better known cause, as soon as the effects are identical. Therefore the pressure on the retina, which is generated by external light, seems to us more familiar than the pressure caused by a hard, non-luminous object. Since pressure is pressure the soul believes* [when perceiving deformation phosphenes] *that light is acting on the retina . . .*' [57, p. 1041]. Haller mentioned the experiments of Morgagni and Langguth and supported the idea that no physical light is generated when the eyeball is deformed [57].

As an example of the discussion on phosphenes in the textbooks of physiology of the early 19th century, we wish to mention *Johann Heinrich Ferdinand Autenrieth*'s '*Handbuch der empirischen Physiologie*' [58]. Autenrieth (1772–1835) taught as professor of medicine at the University of

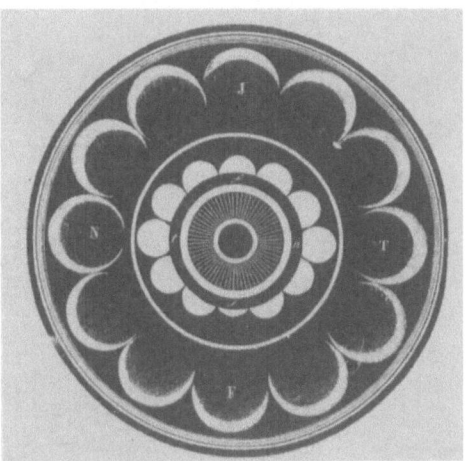

Fig. 6. Serre d'Uzèz published this figure in his '*Essai sur les phosphenes*' [59]. This illustration demonstrates the quarter-moon phosphene which appears at the contralateral side to the indentation site. Serre d'Uzez summarized his observations schematically: The central part of the figure represents the pupil and the iris, the filled circles the site of indentation, the size of these filled circles the strength of local eyeball deformation, and the quarter-moons the phosphene seen in the visual field opposite the respective indentation site.

Tübingen and was one of the protagonists of empirical medicine during the outgoing period of enlightenment and the beginning of romanticism in Germany. In his handbook chapter on vision he also described phosphenes and analysed the light and dark ('*black-bluish*') components of the deformation phosphenes, arguing that the bright parts are caused by retinal excitation, while the dark parts indicate retinal suppression ('*Lähmung*'). Without mentioning Morgagni and Langguth he reported the results of their experiments as proof that no physical light is generated during eyeball deformation [58, Vol. II, p. 191].

The name '*phosphene*' was first coined in 1838 by the French physician *Savigny* [13], and the first extensive review on deformation phosphenes was published in 1853 by the French physiologist *Serre d'Uzèz* [59]. He had also performed detailed experiments on pressure phosphenes in which the relationship between site and strength of eyeball deformation, on the one hand, was carefully determined and on the other, the shape and localization of the phosphene in the visual field. In Fig. 6 his findings are summarized.

One of the leading sensory physiologists of the first half of the 19th century, the Bohemian *Jan Evangelista Pŭrkyne* (1787–1864), professor of physiology at the Prussian University of Breslau (now Wroclaw, Poland) and later at the University of Prague, also conducted extensive investigations on deformation phosphenes [60]. The first study of Pŭrkyne on the

78

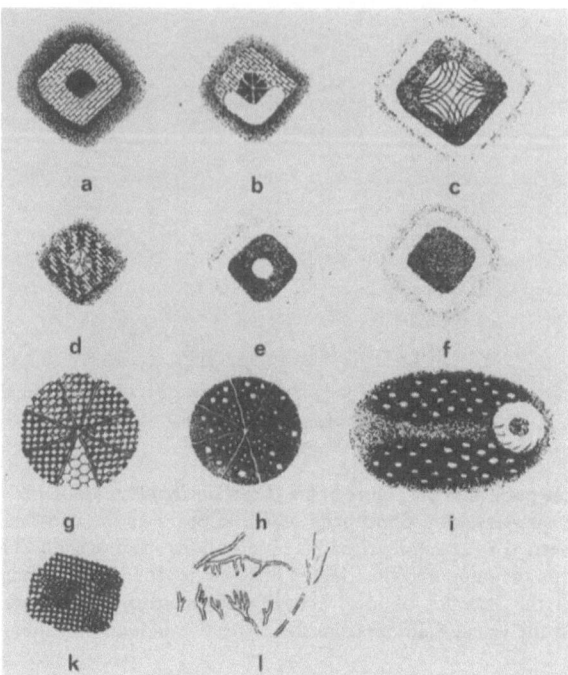

Fig. 7. Selection of deformation phosphenes as observed by J.E. Pŭrkyne [61, 68]. For further explanation see text.

'*Druckfigur des Auges*', as he called them, was published in his doctoral thesis [61]. He described the subjective light sensations evoked by deformation of the eyeball on the side of the cornea. Immediately after the onset of pressure he observed a *ring of light* consisting of small light or dark squares and a round dark hole in the middle. When the pressure was maintained, the hole became filled with bright lines and the size of the ring increased (Fig. 7a–d). Within a few seconds the phenomenon was transformed into a larger ring of light, whereby a luminous central structure became visible (Fig. 7e). As soon as the deforming pressure was released, the central structure disappeared, but the ring was still visible for a few seconds (Fig. 7f). Pŭrkyne noted the variability of the '*Druckfigur*' when he repeated the experiment. In some cases he also observed *patterned visual structures* as shown in Fig. 7g and k and light nebula superimposed by bright stars (Fig. 7h). When the pressure was relieved, he noted fragments of the figure of retinal vessels (Fig. 7l).

In addition to the deformation phosphenes Pŭrkyne also observed short phosphenes during large saccades:

'*If I cover the eye well and move it fast and with some force towards the outer corners of the orbit, a large luminous ring appears on the outer side of the dark field of vision*' [61, p. 26] (Fig. 7i). He concluded that this light is caused by the sudden stretch of the optic nerve, which produces '*in the substance of the nerve electrical antagonistic processes causing the development of light . . .*' [61, p. 27].

In his second book on vision in 1825 Pŭrkyne extended these studies. He described how he could observe weakly illuminated phosphenes of al elliptic shape in a totally dark room when he pressed his eyelids tightly together and then suddenly relaxed them. In contrast to most reports, Pŭrkyne, who was an extremely careful and skilled observer, repeatedly saw *patterned phosphenes* during the deformation of one eye (Fig. 7g and k). Such patterned phosphenes normally are only visible when both eyeballs are deformed simultaneously [l]: A few seconds after binocular eyeball deformation, in addition to the phenomena known from monocular deformation, the patterned phosphene appears. Square-shaped or rhomboid structures in a regular formation and increasing in size from the center of the field of vision to the periphery appear to flicker at about 10 Hz. In between these flickering patterns very bright non-flickering small stars of a slight bluish colour appear together with some small dark bands extending from the center of the visual field radially to the periphery. These binocular deformation phosphenes are shown in Fig. 1e as they appeared to one of the authors (O.-J. G.). We explored this phenomenon in many subjects, most of them inexperienced and uninformed with regard to phosphenes. In all subjects periodic geometrical patterns as shown in Fig. 1e were described but the details of the light-dark patterns varied from subject to subject [62].

We became curious of course as to why Pŭrkyne's reports should deviate from those of most subjects, in which pattern phosphenes only appeared during *binocular* eyeball deformation. The hypothesis was put forward that Pŭrkyne had an amblyopic eye and poor binocular integration [60]. Indeed we could find some biographic evidence that this was the case [63]. Pŭrkyne was therefore very cautious in describing binocular phenomena of vision.

Despite the fact that all physiologists towards the end of the 18th century were in agreement that eyeball deformation only evokes subjective light and not physical light, the belief that efferent light from the eye could illuminate the extrapersonal space lived on in the public mind as well as in the conceptions of some medical doctors. In 1834 Johannes Müller reported on such a case, which was analysed by a *Hofrath Seiler*, specialist in forensic medicine: '*The question whether the human eye can see in the dark due to emission of subjective light was analysed in a forensic medical examination. A dignified priest had been robbed on a dark night by two men and his right eye hit by a stone. "In the same moment light similar to electrical glare or the illumination caused by summer lightning was emitted from his eyes. He could therefore distinctly recognize the culprit." Hofrath Seiler, who was asked to decide on the question, did not directly support this statement, since analogous cases were lacking. However he considered it as a possible argument, because some men and animals can see in the dark (which only proves that they have a sensitive retina). He mentioned by name Kaspar Hauser, who could see at dawn much better than in the daylight. Furthermore, he argued that by pressure on the eye, light sensations are evoked and finally, that in many animals and some men light was observed in the eyes. Seiler himself claimed to have seen the glare in eyes of cats in totally dark cellars, all the brighter, the more excited the animals were by an affect, hunting the prey etc . . .'*

Müller, of course, contradicted this opinion and wrote that Seiler could easily have refuted his hypothesis by going into a dark room, deforming his eye till the deformation phosphenes appeared and then trying to read by the light of these phosphenes. Finally Müller *'regretted that such an illustrious and commendable scholar had in this case supported medical superstition'* [64, p. 140–42].

With the exception of Tyler's study [1] on binocular deformation phosphenes, no new essential discoveries on phosphenes were made after Pŭrkyne, but the mechanisms leading to this curious percept were discussed anew by each generation of physiologists [65, p. 236–241]. During the first decades of the 20th century some sensory physiologists believed deformation phosphenes to be caused by the *increased intraocular pressure* accompanying eyeball deformation and leading to retinal ischemia [66]. Others, such as Stigler [67], maintained the hypothesis that it is primarily the *retinal stretch* which leads to the phenomenon. This idea was also supported by the appearance of accommodation phosphenes [68, 69, 70]: When one looks at an imaginary distant object in total darkness and then directs the eyes as quickly as possible to the tip of the nose, the strong accommodation changes the force transmitted from the ciliary muscle and the elastic lens via the *Zonula Zinnii* fibers to the retina. This stretch leads to a ring-shaped phosphene of mild intensity seen in the outer periphery of the field of vision. Since the intraocular pressure is not essentially changed by such accommodative processes, the retinal stretch hypothesis seemed to be more plausible than that of retinal ischemia or hypoxia. The stretch hypothesis is also supported by the appearance of saccadic phosphenes, repeatedly mentioned above. Saccadic phosphenes are circular or semicircular light sensations located around the projection of the optic nerve in the visual field (observation in total darkness). When the eyes are moved by horizontal saccades to the right, this light ring is seen excentrically on the left side, and when the eyes perform a saccade to the left, the light ring appears on the right side. From this it is concluded that inward movement of the eye stretches the retina near the optic papilla and thus evokes the ring-shaped or half-ring-shaped phosphene. Patients suffering from *optic neuritis* frequently report seeing rather bright saccadic phosphenes. This is presumably caused by the increased sensibility of the swollen optic nerve to retinal stretch and the edema of the papilla.

7. Neurophysiology of deformation phosphenes, a postscript

During the last 15 years we became interested in the neurophysiological basis of deformation phosphenes and consequently performed experiments in anaesthetized cats [51, 71, 72, 73]. By means of tungsten microelectrodes the activity of single *on-center* or *off-center ganglion cells* was recorded from optic tract fibers. These essential results can be summarized in one sentence: *The great majority of on-center ganglion cells*, normally activated when the retina is *illuminated* by light and inhibited when the light is turned off, increased their neuronal activity after a latency of 0.2 to 3 seconds during constant eyeball deformation in total darkness, while the *off-center ganglion cells*, which normally are transiently inhibited by illumination of the retina, were inhibited with a delay of 0.2 to 4 seconds by eyeball deformation. This response scheme and the explanation of deformation activation are shown in Fig. 8.

We interpreted our neurophysiological results by the hypothesis that eyeball deformation leads to retinal stretch, which in turn increases the surface of *horizontal cells*. This surface increase leads to depolarization of the membrane potential of horizontal cells, which then is transmitted to the bipolar cells connected with the horizontal cells. Hereby (as is normally the case when the horizontal cell membrane potential is depolarized), the *on-bipolars*, i.e., the cone on-bipolars in the light-adapted retina and the rod-bipolars in the dark-adapted retina, are depolarized and the *off-bipolars* are hyperpolarized by the depolarization of the synaptic contacts between horizontal cells and bipolar cells. This mechanism induces the activation of on-center ganglion cells and the inhibition of off-center ganglion cells, which corresponds nicely to what the observer perceives in his visual field, provided that one accepts the idea that the information 'brighter' is conveyed by on-center ganglion cell activity and 'darker' by off-center [for details see 55, 73].

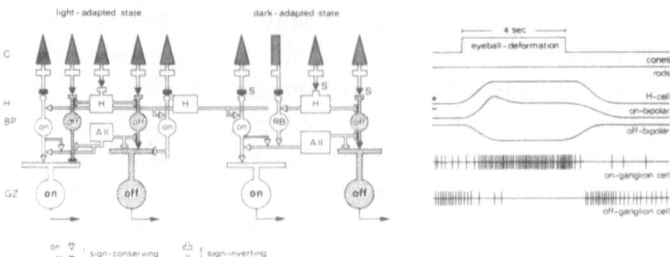

Fig. 8. Scheme of the effect of eyeball deformation on the activity of retinal neurons. The deformation stretches and increases the retinal surface, whereby the horizontal elements in particular (horizontal cells and amacrines) are affected. This leads to an increase in cell surface of these structures and to a *depolarization* of the horizontal cells (H), which in turn causes a depolarization of on-bipolars (BP_{on}) and a hyperpolarization of off-bipolars (BP_{off}). These changes are transmitted to the corresponding ganglion cells (G), which are activated (on-center ganglion cells) or inhibited (off-center ganglion cells). A similar depolarization of the amacrine cells (AII) could also lead to a modification of the ganglion cell responses. Due to their antagonistic innervation of on- and off-ganglion cells, the amacrine type II is a candidate for the mediation of direct stretch responses. The responses of retinal ganglion cells during and after eyeball deformation, however, are dominated by the horizontal cell depolarization. In the dark-adapted retina, the horizontal cell depolarization is mediated through the rod bipolar cells (RB), which activate AII-amacrines, activating in turn on-ganglion cells and inhibiting off-ganglion cells. Excitatory ('sign-conserving') synapses are drawn as arrows, inhibitory ('sign-reversing') synapses as bars. When the *rod-amacrine* cell is directly depolarized by deformation, this depolarization would also lead to an activation of on-ganglion cells and an inhibition of off-ganglion cells, since the synaptic endings of the rod-amacrine cell are functionally not uniform and have a 'polar' organisation.

Acknowledgement

The work was supported in part by grants of the Deutsche Forschungs-gemeinschaft (Gr 161, Ha 1499-1). We thank Mrs. Elisabeth Vesper for her help in searching out literature and Mrs. Judith Dames for the correction of the English text. The senior author (O.-J.G.) gratefully acknowledges the support by an Akademiestipendium of the Volkswagen Foundation.

References

1. Tyler Ch. Some new entoptic phenomena. Vision Res 1978; 18: 1633–1639.
2. Theophrast of Eresos. Theophrastus and the Greek physiological psychology before Aristotle. 'De sensu' transl. by Stratton GM, London: G. Allen and Unwin, 1917. Reprint Amsterdam: E.J. Bonset 1964; 227 p; quoted in text as DS.
3. Diels H, Kranz W. Die Fragmente der Vorsokratiker, Vol. I. Basel: Weidmann, 1951; 504 p.
4. Aristoteles. Über die Sinneswahrnehmung und ihre Gegenstände ('De sensu et sensato'). In: Gohlke P, ed. and transl. Die Lehrschriften, Vol. VI/2: Kleine Schriften zur Seelenkunde, 2nd edn. Paderborn: Schöningh, 1953; 22–61.

5. Platon. Timaios. In: Loewenthal E, ed. Platon, Sämtliche Werke, Vol. III. Köln, Olten: Hegner, 1969; 93–191.

6. Hirschberg J. Geschichte der Augenheilkunde. I: Geschichte der Augenheilkunde im Altertum. In: Graefe-Saemisch, Handbuch der gesammten Augenheilkunde, Vol. XII/2. Leipzig: Engelmann, 1899; 419 p.

7. Diogenes Laertius. Leben und Meinungen berühmter Philosophen. Transl. by Appelt O. Reich K, ed. 2nd edn. Hamburg: Meiner, 1967; 411 p.

8. Arnold EV. Roman Stoicism. (Reprint Freeport, New York: Books for Libraries Press, 1971; 478 p.) 1911.

9. Watson G. The Stoic theory of knowledge. Oxford: Vincent Baxter, 1966; 106 p.

10. Epikur. Philosophie der Freude. Mewaldt J, ed. Stuttgart: Kröner, 1973; 95 p.

11. Katz O. Die Augenanatomie des Galenos. Erster (theoretischer) Teil: Über Anatomie und Physiologie des Sehorgans. Medical Dissertation, University of Berlin, 1890; 126 p.

12. Siegel RE. Galen on Sense Perception. Basel: Karger, 1970; 216 p.

13. Hagner M. Zur Geschichte vom Licht im Auge und der Physiologie des Druckphosphens im Verhältnis zu den jeweils zeitgenössischen Sehtheorien. Medical Dissertation, Freie Universität Berlin, 1987; 164 p.

14. Lindberg DC. Theories of Vision from Al-Kindi to Kepler. Chicago: The University of Chicago Press, 1976; 304 p.

15. Meyerhof M, Prüfer C. Die Augenanatomie des Hunain b. Ishaq. Sudhoffs Arch Gesch Med 1910; 4: 163–90.

16. Meyerhof M, Prüfer C. Die Lehre von Sehen bei Humain b. Ishaq. Sudhoffs Arch. Gesch. Med. 1911; 5: 21–38.

17. Alhazen. De Aspectibus. In: Risner F, ed. Opticae thesaurus Alhazeni arabis libri septem. 1572 Basel: Per Episcopios. Reprint with an introduction by D. Lindberg. New York: Johnson Reprint Corporation, 1972; 288 p.

18. Bauer H. Die Psychologie Alhazens auf Grund von Alhazens Optik. Beiträge zur Geschichte der Philosophie des Mittelalters, Vol. X, Fasc. 5. Münster: Aschendorff, 1911; 72 p.

19. Schramm M. Zur Entwicklung der physiologischen Optik in der arabischen Literatur. Sudhoffs Arch Gesch Med 1959; 43: 289–316.

20. Russell GA. The emergence of physiological optics. In: Morelon R, Rashed R, eds. Science in Islamic Civilisation. London: Crom Helm, 1990 (in press).

21. Wiedemann E. Ibn Sinas Anschauung vom Sehvorgang. Arch Gesch Naturw u Technik 1913; 4: 239–241.

22. Hirschberg J, Lippert J. Die Augenheilkunde des Avicenna. Translation from the arabic text. Leipzig: Engelmann, 1902.

23. Baur L. Die philosophischen Werke des Robert Grosseteste. Beiträge zur Geschichte der Philosophie des Mittelalters, Vol. IX. Münster: Aschendorff, 1912.

24. Bacon R. The opus majus of Roger Bacon, Vol II. Bridges JH, ed. London (Reprint Frankfurt: Minerva, 1964) 1900.

25. Albertus Magnus. Summae de creaturis. In: Borgnet A, ed. Opera omnia, Vol XXXV. Paris, 1890–1899.

26. Cusanus N. Compendium (Kurze Darstellung der philosophisch-theologischen Lehre). Lateinisch-Deutsch. Hamburg: F. Meiner, 1982; 110 p.

27. Cusanus N. Schrift vom Geist (Liber de mente). Transl. by H. Cassirer. In: Cassirer E. Individuum und Kosmos in der Philosophie der Renaissance. Darmstadt: Wissenschaftliche Buchgesellschaft, 1977; 202–300.

28. Fabricius ab Aquapendente H. 'De actione oculorum, pars secunda'. In: Opera omnia anatomica et physiologica. Leipzig: J.F. Gleditsch, 1687; 452 p.

29. Koelbing H. Il Trattato 'De visione' di Girolamo Fabrici d'Acquapendente (Venezia 1600). Atti del XXXIII Congresso nazionale della Società Italiana de Storia della Medicina. Padua: La Garangola, 1985; 29–33.
30. Plater F. De corporis humani structura et usu. Basel: Froben, 1583; 197 p.
31. Koelbing H. Renassance der Augenheilkunde 1540–1630. Bern, Stuttgart: Huber, 1967; 198 p.
32. Bauhin C. Deo corporis humani fabrica, Libri IV. Basel: Frobenius, 1590.
33. Bauhin C. Theatrum anatomicum. Frankfurt a.M.: Becker, 1605; 1340 p.
34. Koelbing H. Kepler und die physiologische Optik. Sein Beitrag und seine Wirkung. In: Krafft F, Meyer K, Sticker B, eds. Internationales Kepler-Symposion. Weil der Stadt 1971. Hildesheim: Gerstenberg, 1973; 229–45.
35. Kepler J. Ad Vitelloni paralipomena, quibus astronomiae pars optica traditur. Frankfurt 1604. In: Hammer F, ed. Gesammelte Werke, Vol. II. München: Beck, 1939.
36. Kepler J. Dioptrice. Augsburg: Frank, 1611. In: von Dyck W, Casper M, eds. Gesammelte Werke, Vol IV, München: Beck, 1937–1964.
37. Kepler J. Johannes Keplers Behandlung des Sehens. Trans. by Plehn F. Zeitschrift für ophthalmologische Optik mit Einschluß der Instrumentenkunde, 1920–21; 8: 154–57; 9: 13–26, 40–54, 73–87, 103–09, 143–52, 177–82.
38. Scheiner C. Oculus: Hoc est: Fundamentum opticum. 1st edn. (1619); Innsbruck: Agricola, 1648.
39. Plempius VF. Ophthalmographia sive tractatio de oculi fabrica, actione et usu. Amsterdam: Laurentius, 1632; 340 p.
40. Lindeboom GA. Descartes and Medicine. Amsterdam: Rodopi, 1978; 134 p.
41. Descartes R. Dioptrique. In: Adam C, Tannery P, eds. Oeuvres de Descartes, Vol. VI. Paris, 1897–1913.
42. Descartes R. Traité de l'homme, 1664. Germ. transl. by: Rothschuh K, 'Über den Menschen' (1632) sowie 'Beschreibung des menschlichen Körpers (1648). Heidelberg: Schneider, 1969; 202 p.
43. Ferrero N. Leonardo da Vinci: of the eye. Amer J Ophthalmol 1952; 35: 507–521.
44. Boyle R. The experimental history of colours begun, 1st edn. In: The Works of Robert Boyle, Vol. 1. (Reprint Hildesheim: Olms 1965) London, 1664; p. 668 ff.
45. Henninius HCh. Johannis Claubergi Vita. In: Clauberg J. Opera omnia philosophica, Vol I. Amsterdam: Janson-Waesberg, 1691; 1–15.
46. Clauberg J. Theoria corporum viventium. In: Opera omnia philosophica, Vol I. (Reprint Hildesheim: Olms, 1968) Amsterdam: Janson-Waesberg, 1664; 163–208.
47. Malebranche N. Entretiens sur la métaphysique et sur la religion. In: Robinet A, ed. Oeuvres de Malebranche. Vol. XIII. Paris: J. Vrin, Librairie Philosophique, 1965.
48. Bartholinus Th. De luce hominum et brutorum, Libri III. Copenhagen: Godiccaen, 1669; 531 p.
49. Briggs W. Ophthalmo-graphia sive oculi eiusque partium descriptio anatomica. Cambridge: Hyes, 1676; 80 p.
50. Newton I. Opticks. Or, a treatise of the reflections, refractions, inflections and colours of light. London, 1730. Reprint New York: Dover Edition, 4th edn, 1952; 406 p.
51. Morgagni GB. Adversaria Anatomica Omnia. Padua, 1719; 2nd edn. Leyden 1741.
52. Langguth GA. De luce ex pressione oculi. Wittenberg: E.G. Eichsfeld, 1742; 16 p.
53. Morgagni GB. De sedibus et causis morborum. 2 Vol. Venice: Remondian, 1761.
54. Morgagni GB. Von dem Sitze und den Ursachen der Krankheiten. Vol. I: Krankheiten des Kopfes. Altenburg, 1771.
55. Grüsser O-J, Hagner M, Przybyszewski A. The effect of dark adaptation on the responses of cat retinal ganglion cells to eyeball deformation. Vision Res 1989; 29: 1059–1068.

56. Boerhaave H. Kurze, doch gründliche Abhandlungen von Augenkrankheiten und derselben Cur. Transl. by Clauder GF. Nürnberg: Schwarzkopf, 1759; 310 p.
57. Haller A von. Anfangsgründe der Physiologie des menschlichen Körpers, Vol. V. Transl. from the Latin by J.S. Hallen. 1768; Berlin: Voss.
58. Autenrieth JHF. Handbuch der empirischen menschlichen Physiologie, 3 Vols. Tübingen: Heerbrandt, 1802/1803; 396 p.
59. Serre d'Uzèz. Essai sur les phosphènes ou anneaux lumineux de la rétine. Paris: Masson, 1853.
60. Grüsser O-J. Pŭrkyne's contribution to the physiology of the visual, vestibular and the oculomotor system. Hum Neurobiol 1984; 3: 129–144.
61. Purkinje JE. Beyträge zur Kenntniss des Sehens in subjectiver Hinsicht. Prag: Calve, 1819; 109 p.
62. Müller J. Psychologische Diplomarbeit, Physiologisches Institut, Freie Universität Berlin, 1985.
63. Tschermak-Seyssenegg A von. Joh. Ev. Pŭrkyne als ein Begründer des exakten Subjectivismus. In: In Memoriam Joh. Ev. Pŭrkyne 1787–1937. Prag, 1937; 76–96.
64. Müller J. Jahresbericht über die Fortschritte der anatomisch-physiologischen Wissenschaften im Jahre 1833. Archiv für Anatomie, Physiologie und Wissenschaftliche Medicin, Berlin, 1834.
65. Helmholtz H von. Handbuch der physiologischen Optik. Hamburg und Leipzig: Voss, 1896; 1334 p.
66. Ebbecke U. Entoptische Versuche über Netzhautdurchblutung. Pflügers Arch 1921; 186: 220–237.
67. Stigler R. Beiträge zur Kenntnis des Druckphosphens. Pflügers Arch 1906; 115: 248–272.
68. Purkinje JE. Beobachtungen und Versuche zur Physiologie der Sinne. II. Neue Beyträge zur Kenntniss des Sehens in subjectiver Hinsicht. Berlin: Reimer, 1825; 191 p.
69. Czermak J. Ueber das Accommodationsphosphen. Graefes Arch ges Ophthalmol 1858; 7: 147–154.
70. Berlin E. Ueber das Accommodationsphosphen. Graefes Arch ges Ophthalmol 1874; 20: 89–97.
71. Grüsser O-J, Grüsser-Cornehls U, Müller J. Neurophysiologische Grundlagen des Druckphosphens. In: Herzau V ed. Pathophysiologie des Sehens, Stuttgart: Enke, 1984; 21–37.
72. Grüsser O-J, Grüsser-Cornehls U, Schreiter U. Responses of cat retinal ganglion cells to eyeball deformation. A neurophysiological basis for pressure phosphenes. In: Maffei L ed. Pathophysiology of the Visual System, The Hague: Junk, 1981; 36–52.
73. Grüsser O-J, Grüsser-Cornehls U, Kusel R, Przybyszewski A. Responses of retinal ganglion cells to eyeball deformation: A neurophysiological basis for pressure phosphenes. Vision Res 1989; 29: 181–194.
74. Grüsser O-J. Interaction of efferent and afferent signals in visual perception. A history of ideas and experimental paradigms. Acta Psychol 1986; 63: 3–21.
75. Galen C. On the Usefulness of the Parts, 2 Vol. May MT, ed. and transl. Ithaca, 1968.

Address for correspondence: Dr O.J. Grüsser, Dept. of Physiology, Arnimallee 22, 1 Berlin 33 (West), FRG.

Documenta Ophthalmologica **74**: 87–93, 1990.
© 1990 *Kluwer Academic Publishers.*

Antonie Cramer's explanation of accommodation

I. DEN TONKELAAR, H.E. HENKES & G.K. VAN LEERSUM
F.C. Donders Institute of Ophthalmology, Utrecht, The Netherlands

Abstract. In the middle of the last century the question of the origin of accommodation was still unsolved. At the suggestion of Donders, Cramer used in 1851 a microscope to demonstrate that accommodation has to be ascribed to an increase in the curvature of the lens. Donders himself had several instruments made for the same purpose. These are still present in the collection of the Royal Netherlands Ophthalmic Hospital.

From 1842 to 1848 F.C. Donders (1818–1889) earned a living as a teacher in anatomy, physiology and histology at the Utrecht military medical academy. His salary of 800 guilders a year, however, was hardly enough to maintain his wife and child. A welcome supplement to his income was provided by his translation activities. Donders' Dutch translation of Ruete's 'Lehrbuch der Ophthalmologie' was published in 1846. This work stimulated him to start his own research in ophthalmology [1, 2]. While he worked at the translation, he had already developed his own views on certain subjects as we can learn from the many annotations he added to the translation. The most extensive annotation was made to Ruete's assertion that accommodation is due to a displacement of the lens [3]. Donders' criticism refered to the fact that Ruete tried to answer a physiological problem with a subjective opinion, without the support of objective observations. From this kind of criticism we recognise Donders' scientific conception as well as that of his teacher Schroeder van der Kolk, the Utrecht professor of physiology. The latter took up the question of accommodation, suggesting in 1848 to the 'Hollandsche Maatschappij der Wetenschappen' (Dutch Society of Sciences), to offer a prize for the best treatise on the mechanism of accommodation [4].

Donders did not compete in the contest, but the problem kept him busy. In 1848 he was already on the right track, without realising it however. In that year he wrote a paper about Sanson's test (testing the opacity of the lens using the reflecting images of Purkinje, especially the reflecting image of the posterior surface of the lens [5]. In his paper Donders gave useful instructions how one could more easily observe Purkinje's images. At that moment Donders did not take the step that studying the reflecting images could

88

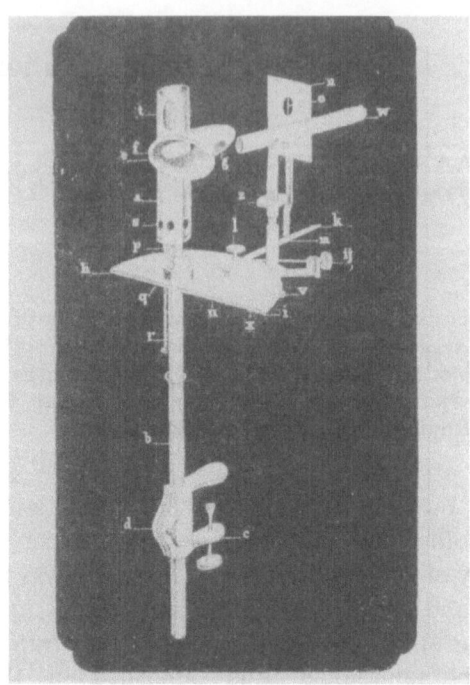

Fig. 1. Instrument designed by Cramer (1851) by means of which he demonstrated for the first time that accommodation for the first time that accommodation is due to a change in the shape of the lens. The subject's eye is at position *e*; a candle light (behind opening *t*) shines through the hole *f*; the observer is at position *w* and studies the reflecting images with the microscope (tube *w*) via opening *g*; the subject first looks at thread *o* and next in the distance without changing the direction of the visual axis.

produce information about changes in the shape of the lens. It did not take long before Maximilian Langenbeck in 1849 discussed the application of the reflecting images in the study of accommodation. This subject was somewhat hidden among a variety of subjects in Langenbeck's book on surgery and ophthalmology [6]. When Donders came across the book by coincidence, he immediately reported Langenbeck's findings in the 'Nederlandsch Lancet', a Dutch journal of which he was one of the editors. Langenbeck studied the relation between the reflection images at different distances of fixation of the eye. With the naked eye however, he was unable to decide about changes in diameter of the reflecting images. The angle of incidence of the light he used in his studies was very unfavourable to get reliable results [7]. Langenbeck concluded nevertheless that during accommodation the anterior surface of the lens becomes more convex. Donders could not confirm Langenbeck's observations. However, he expected to get results when both the distance and the diameter of the reflecting images

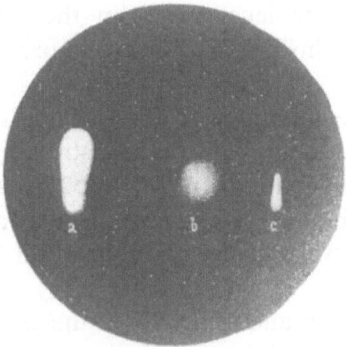

Fig. 2a. Reflecting images of a) cornea b) anterior surface c) posterior surface during accommodation, while fixating thread *o*.

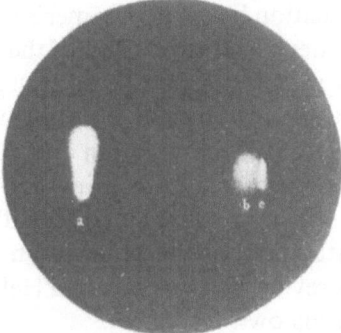

Fig. 2b. Reflecting images of a) cornea b) anterior surface c) posterior surface while fixating a distant point.

could be studied by means of a microscope [8]. Together with his friend and physicist van Rees, Donders made some efforts in this direction, but he didn't succeed [9].

The idea of using a microscope, however was successfully adopted by Antonie Cramer in Groningen. He was a doctor medicinae et chirurgicae et obstetricae with a poor health and for that reason not fit for a profession in surgery. He compensated this drawback by devoting himself to scientific research [10]. Notwithstanding his weak constitution his perseverance was sufficient to solve the problem of the origin of accommodation.

He had an instrument, named ophthalmoscope, made by the Groningen instrumentmaker Deutgen (Fig. 1) [7]. Cramer studied the reflecting images of a. the cornea b. the anterior surface of the lens and c. the posterior surface of the lens, while fixating a stretched thread nearby (Fig. 2a) and at a distance (Fig. 2b). He concluded from the displacement of the image b. of

90

the anterior surface of the lens and from the increased diameter and decreased lucidity of this image, that the curvature of the lens increases at accommodation.

In November 1851 he submitted to the 'Hollandsche Maatschappij der Wetenschappen' a treatise together with the instrument he used as an answer to the forementioned competition. In May 1852 his answer was awarded a gold medal and a premium of 150 guilders. The award of a premium was quite exceptional.[1] However Cramer had to wait till 1853 to see his treatise printed [7].

Independently of Cramer, and using almost the same methods, Helmholtz came to identical results, which he communicated to the Berlin Academy of Sciences in February 1853. This was before Cramer's treatise had been published! [9].

Thanks to Donders' attention however, Cramer's priority was warranted. In a paper titled 'de stand der iris' (the position of the iris) published in 1851 [11] Cramer had casually mentioned that he had succeeded to determine a change in the shape of the lens at accommodation. Donders was immediately aware of the importance of this observation and devoted a special paper to the subject in the 'Nederlandsch Lancet' in 1851–1852 [12]. When the 'Hollandsche Maatschappij der Wetenschappen' finally published Cramer's treatise, Donders paid attention to the publication by means of a book review of 40 pages.[2] In his review he also discussed Helmholtz's observations as well as communicated his own results [9].

Donders, namely, had an instrument made by the Amsterdam instrumentmaker Epkens (Fig. 3). With this instrument even the amount of displacement of the anterior surface of the lens at accommodation could be measured. Moreover Donders intended to investigate in particular the position of the posterior surface of the lens [13], as Cramer had mentioned that neither the position, nor the curvature of the posterior surface changed. In 1855 Helmholtz demonstrated that the curvature of the posterior surface also increases [14].

It was not permitted for Cramer to do any further research in accommodation. He died 32 years old on the first of January 1855 [10, 15].

Donders continued his investigations. He had two more instruments built by Epkens with which he could measure the curvature of the lens more accurately (Fig. 4 and Fig. 5) [16]. He named these instruments 'phacoidoscoop' [16, 17]. In 1864 Donders described one of these instruments in his famous book 'On the Anomalies of Accommodation and

[1] Mr. de Bruyn, adjunct secretary of the Dutch Society of Sciences (pers. comm.).
[2] Nederlandsch Lancet, 1853–1854.

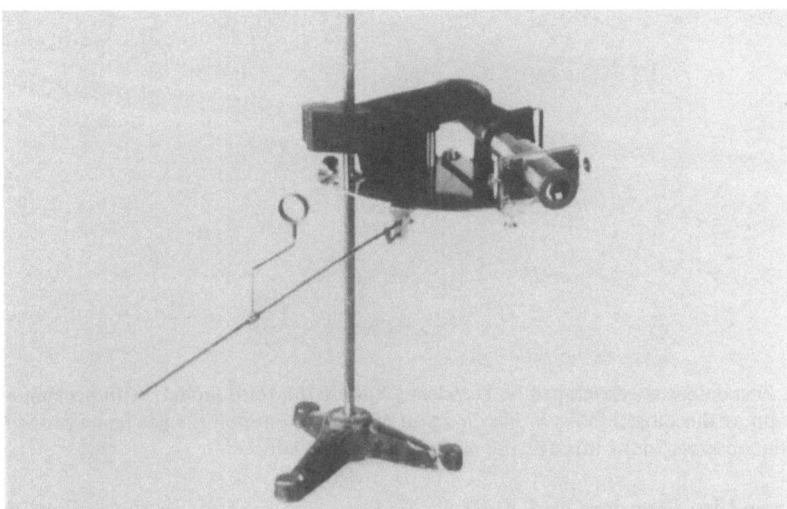

Fig. 3. Phacoidoscope designed by Donders (1853); first model. The subject's eye is at the corner and looks in the direction of the fixation point. The light is placed at the side of the eye at the other end of the tube and illuminates the eye by means of a mirror; the observer studies the eye with a microscope.

Refraction of the Eye' [16]. The illustration of the instrument however is very schematic and could depict either model 2 or 3. In 1876 Donders also sent a phacoidoscope (most probably the third model) to the Loan Exhibition of Scientific Apparatus in London [18]. All three instruments

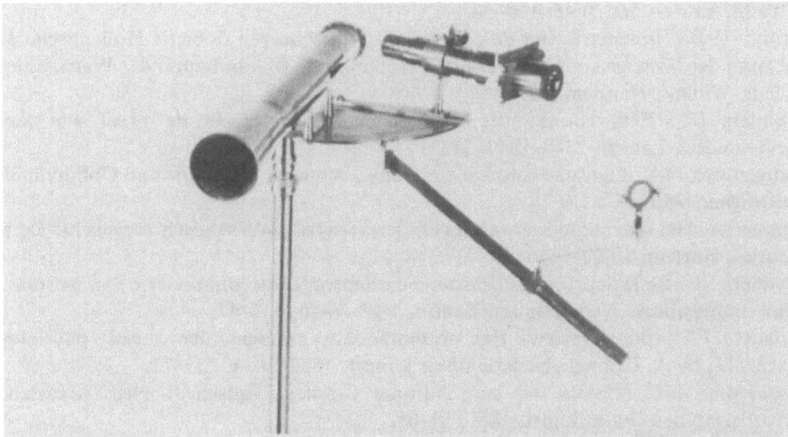

Fig. 4. Phacoidoscope developed by Donders (1864); second model. The subject's eye is at the corner; the light is placed at the wide opening of the illumination tube and the observer looks through the microscope on the right.

92

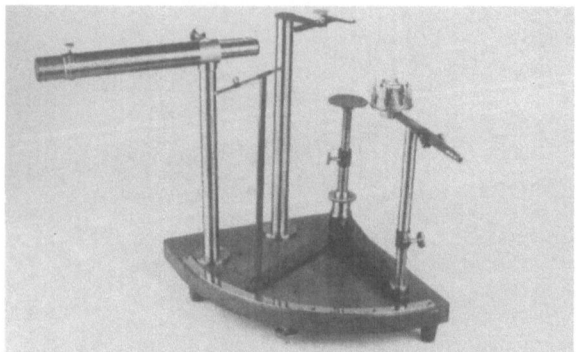

Fig. 5. Phacoidoscope developed by Donders (1864–1876), third model. With his chin on the chin support the subject looks in the direction of the fixation point; a gas flame provides the light; the observer looks through the microscope at the left.

developed by Donders and built by Epkens are present in the collection of the Royal Netherlands Ophthalmic Hospital.[3] The original instrument used by Cramer could not be traced despite an intensive search throughout the Netherlands.

References

1. Hirschberg J. Graefe-Saemisch, Handbuch der Gesammten Augenheilkunde. Julius Springer Verlag, Berlin, 1918, XV Bd. Abt. 1, Par. 1039, p. 178.
2. Leersum van EC. Het levenswerk van F.C. Donders. Bohn, Haarlem, 1932.
3. Ruete CGT. Leerboek der Ophthalmologie. Translated by Donders. van der Post, Utrecht/Amsterdam, 1846; 120–24.
4. Bruijn de JG. Inventaris van de prijsvragen uitgeschreven door de Hollandsche Maatschappij der Wetenscappen, 1753–1917. Hollandsche Maatschappij der Wetenschappen, Tjeenk Willink, Haarlem, 1977.
5. Donders FC. Een woord over de aanwendingswijze van de proef van Sanson. Nederlandsch Lancet, 1848–1849; 211–17.
6. Langenbeck MA. Klinische beiträge aus dem Gebiete der Chirurgie und Ophthalmologie, Göttingen, 1849.
7. Cramer A. Het accommodatievermogen dere oogen physiologisch toegelicht. De erven Loosjes, Harlem, 1853.
8. Donders FC. Reflexieproef van Purkinje en Sanson en accommodatie van het oog naar Max. Langenbeck. Nederlandsch Lancet, 1849–1850; 132–47.
9. Donders FC. (book review) Het accommodatievermogen der oogen, physiologisch toegelicht, by A. Cramer. Nederlandsch Lancet, 1853–1854, 235–73.
10. Swaagman AH. Herinnering aan Antonie Cramer. Tijdschrift Ned. Maatsch. tot bevordering der Geneeskunst, 1855; 54–64.
11. Cramer A. Mededeelingen uit het gebied der Ophthalmologie. Tijdschrfit Ned. Maatsch. tot bevordering der Geneeskunst, 1851; 99–119.

[3] The temporary address of the collection is Plompetorengracht 9–11, NL-3512 CA, Utrecht.

12. Donders FC. Cramers ontdekking van den grond des accommodatievermogens van het oog. Nederlandsch Lancet, 1851-1852; 529-32.

13. Versl. K.A.v.W. Dll, 1853; 308.

14. Helmholtz H. Ueber die Accommodation des Auges. Archiv für Ophthalmologie, herausgegeben von Arlt, Donders und von Graefe, I Bd, Abt. 2, 1855; 1-74.

15. Molhuysen PC, Blok PJ. Nieuw Nederlands Biografisch Woordenboek IV. Sythoff, Leiden, 1918; 466.

16. Donders FC. On the anomalies of accommodation and refraction of the eye. The New Sydenham Society, London, 1864; 10-19.

17. Donders FC. Ametropie en hare gevolgen. Jaarlijksch Verslag betrekkelijk de verpleging en het onderwijs in het Nederlandsch Gasthuis voor Ooglijders, 1, Wetenschappelijke bijbladen (yearly report concerning nursing and education in the Netherlands Ophthalmic Hospital, Scientific suppl). ed.: F.C. Donders, Van de Weijer, Utrecht, 1860; 73-86.

18. Donders FC. Korte beschrijving van alhier geconstrueerde werktuigen. Jaarlijksch Verslag betrekkelijk de verpleging en het onderwijs in het Nederlandsch Gasthuis voor Ooglijders, 18, Wetenschappelijke bijbladen. ed.: F.C. Donders, Van de Weijer, Utrecht, 1877; 63-76.

Address for correspondence: I. den Tonkelaar, F.C. Donders Inst. of Ophthalmology, P.O. Box 85.500, 3508 GA Utrecht, The Netherlands.

Documenta Ophthalmologica **74**: 95–112, 1990.
© 1990 *Kluwer Academic Publishers.*

19th Century mechanical models of eye movements, Donders' law, Listing's law and Helmholtz' direction circles

H.J. SIMONSZ[1] & I. DEN TONKELAAR[2]
[1] *Netherlands Ophthalmic Research Institute, Amsterdam, The Netherlands**
[2] *Keeper, Ophthalmic Collection of the former Royal Netherlands Ophthalmic Hospital*

Key words: Listing's law, Donders' law, pseudotorsion, ocular counterrolling, ophthalmotropes

Abstract. Donders, Ruete, von Graefe, von Helmholtz, Listing, Volkmann and many others have provided the broad outline of an answer to the question how the eye rotates during eye movements. Many mechanical models of eye movements, ophthalmotropes, have been constructed and studied in the nineteenth century. These models have primarily served to explain Donders' and Listing's Laws on the nature of eye movements. As both Donders' Law and Listing's Law are easier to understand when seen against the background of the coordinate systems used to describe eye movements, all of the coordinate systems currently in use in the diagnosis and treatment of strabismus are described. In addition, the reader is introduced to a coordinate system based on von Helmholtz' direction circles, circles describing the direction of the horizontal and vertical retinal meridians in all positions of gaze.

Donder's Law

'De werking en verrigting der oogspieren behoort tot die onderwerpen, welke door physiologen ten allen tijde met ijver en een zekere voorliefde zijn behandeld, en deze ijver vond in de voor eenige jaren zooveel gerucht makende operatiën tegen het scheelzien en de bijziendheid overvloedig voedsel.' (The action and effect of eye muscles is one of the subjects that have always been treated by physiologists with zeal and predilection, and this zeal has been nourished by the operations for squint and for myopia that caused so much uproar some years ago.) This first sentence of F.C. Donders' first article on eye muscle mechanics applied in 1846 as it applies today. Donders, Ruete, von Graefe, von Helmholtz, Listing, Volkmann and many others have provided the broad outline of an answer to the question how the eye rotates during eye movements. Donders had become interested in eye movements when he translated Professor C.G.T. Ruete's 'Lehrbuch der Ophthalmologie' (1846). He was a young doctor in the military in Utrecht, earned 800 guilders a year and, hence, did translation work to earn extra money.

*This article is part of a thesis submitted to the University of Giessen (Simonsz, 1990).

Ruete (1845) had developed in Scharmbeck the first mechanical model of the eye and its muscles. He called it an 'ophthalmotrope'.

Ruete also studied the rotation of his own eye about the visual axis. He was able to observe the rotation of his own eye about the visual axis by using an afterimage with the form of a + cross. A green afterimage was produced by looking at a red cross for a long time. He then looked at a screen in front of him to see whether the afterimage remained vertical when he looked right, left, up or down. Donders repeated these experiments and found that the afterimage cross tilted, when he looked in tertiary positions of gaze (i.e. right-up, right-down, left-up or left-down): He found that the amount of torsion depended upon the amount of elevation or depression and right or left gaze (Donders' Law).

In 1848 a German edition of Donders' work appeared which drew von Helmholtz' attention. He was very enthusiastic about Donders' discovery and proposed to call the definition of pseudotorsion 'Donders' law'. The reason for the tilt had not been recognized by Donders, however, it was von Helmholtz who explained the reason for pseudotorsion.

The reason for pseudotorsion

Pseudotorsion is caused by the fact that, in tertiary positions of gaze, the vertical retina meridian does not coincide with a vertical line in space, nor does the horizontal retina meridian coincide with a horizontal line in space. The reason for this discrepancy is that horizontal and vertical are defined according to the coordinate system used. To illustrate this point: If the reader is sitting in front of one of the four walls of the room he is in, let him for a moment look at the left upper hand corner of this wall. The reader will perceive the left upper hand 90-degree corner of a wall in front of him as being larger than 90 deg. What, in this case, is horizontal and what is vertical? It is clear that the angle between the horizontal and the vertical retinal meridians is perceived as 90 degrees at all times, no matter what the direction of gaze is. Hence, the afterimage cross cannot coincide with the left upperhand corner of the wall in front of us. The rays of the left upper hand corner are horizontal and vertical in space but, as the angle is perceived as larger than 90 degrees, the rays of the angle cannot possibly coincide with horizontal and vertical retina meridians. In fact, both rays of the angle, projected on the retina, deviate with a small angle from the horizontal and vertical retinal meridian, one clockwise and one anticlockwise. This small angle is called pseudotorsion.

Summarizing, pseudotorsion results from the coordinate system employed or, in other words the reference that one chooses to be vertical or horizontal (Roelofs 1934, 1954).

The polar coordinate system and Listing's Law

The only coordinate system for describing eye rotations that does not have these flaws is the polar coordinate system. In a polar coordinate system the position of the eye is also determined by two angles: One angle defines the direction of eye movement out of the primary position and a second angle defines the angle of eye movement out of the primary position. In this coordinate system, all tertiary positions of gaze are reached by simple rotation about a single axis. This principle was invented by Professor J.B. Listing, a good friend of Professor Ruete, who had participated with Ruete in the Göttinger Studien with a booklet on entoptic phenomena and cataract (1845).

Ruete (1853) therefore called this principle Listing's Law: 'Aus der oben angegebenen normalen Stellung (Anfangsstellung, Primärstellung) des Auges wird das Auge in irgend eine andere, secundäre, durch die Cooperation der sechs Muskeln in der Weise versetzt, dass man sich diese Versetzung als das Resultat einer Drehung um eine bestimmte Drehungsaxe vorstellen kann, welche jederzeit, durch das Augencentrum gehend, auf der primären und secundären Richtung der optischen Axe zugleich senkrecht steht, so dass also jede secundäre Stellung des Auges zur primären in der Relation steht, vermöge welcher die auf die optische Axe projicirte Drehung = O wird. Diesem Princip zufolge lässt sich aus der bekannten Lage der drei auf je zwei antagonistische Muskeln bezüglichen Drehungsaxen für jede gegebene Secundärstellung des Auges der Wirkungsbetrag jedes Muskels, d.i. die Grösse seiner Verkürzung durch Rechnung bestimmen. Unter den vielfachen Consequenzen dieses Princips verdient die hervorgehoben zu werden, dass nämlich das Auge beim Uebergange aus einer secundären Stellung in eine andere eine ihrer Grösse nach bestimmbare Drehung um seine optische Axe erfährt, welche nur in dem besonderen Fall null ist, wenn die drei Richtungen der optischen Axe in der primären und in den beiden secundären Stellung in einer Ebene liegen' (in short, all secondary and tertiary positions of gaze can be reached by rotation about a single axis that is perpendicular to the primary position of gaze and to the new position of gaze . . . Among the many consequences of this principle, one needs particular emphasis, namely, that the eye will rotate about its optical axis in eye movements from one tertiary to another tertiary position of gaze, this rotation being zero only when the two tertiary positions of gaze and the primary position of gaze are all in a single plane.)

The Ophthalmic Collection of the former Royal Netherlands Ophthalmic Hospital has a copper model that illustrates this principle beautifully (Fig. 1). The name of the place of manufacture, Halle, is engraved in the model.

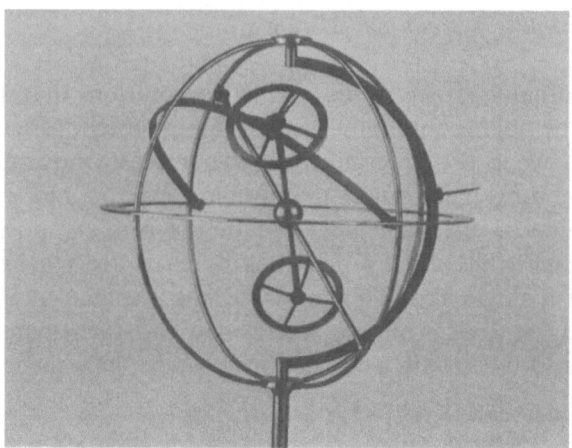

Fig. 1. Ophthalmotrope from the Ophthalmologic Collection of the former Royal Netherlands Ophthalmic Hospital in Utrecht, probably sent by Ruete to Donders ($\pm$ 1852),
demonstrating Donders' and Listing's Laws: all secondary and tertiary positions of gaze can
be reached by rotation about a single axis that is perpendicular to the primary position of gaze
and to the new position of gaze. The primary position of gaze is at the left in the figure. The
eye is represented by a small globe in the center of the model. Two wheels with spokes
(representing the horizontal and vertical retina meridians) are mounted on the tips of an axis
representing the position of gaze. This position-of-gaze axis can tilt about the oblique axis
representing an axis in Listing's plane. At the front of the model (left in the picture) an arc
representing a horizontal meridian in space can be tilted upward: one can see that the
horizontal retina meridian is tilted relative to the meridian arc (Donders' pseudotorsion). At
the back of the model, a vertical arc, representing a vertical meridian in space, can be turned
together with the second spoked wheel: Donders' pseudotorsion is found to occur in the
opposite direction. The horizontal and vertical arc meridians correspond to the way straight
horizontal and vertical lines in space are perceived by the eye in the center of the model: In
the experiments of Donders, he compared horizontal and vertical retina meridians with
horizontal and vertical lines on a wall in front of him, these are represented in this model by
the meridian arcs.

Halle is about 30 km from Leipzig, so it was probably Ruete who sent this
model to Donders.

In Ruete's first ophthalmotrope (1845) the model eye was suspended in
gimbals, i.e. the model eye rotated in a ring that itself could rotate about an
axis that was perpendicular to the first axis, this method of suspension
having been invented by Cardano in the sixteenth century. An improved
version of his ophthalmotrope, presented by him in Leipzig in 1857, no
longer employed suspension with gimbals. The globe was simply pulled
against a ring with screws by the 'muscles'. It can now be seen why Ruete
did not employ a gimbal suspension in the second version of his ophthalmotrope: this kind of globe suspension will not bring the eye in a tertiary
position that complies with Listing's Law: Pseudotorsion will occur in

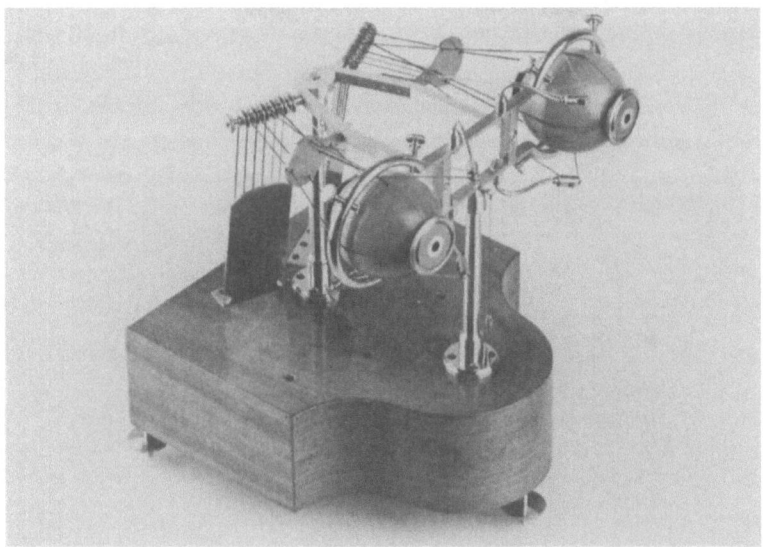

Fig. 2. Ruete's second ophthalmotrope. Note that the eyes are not suspended in gimbals like in Ruete's first ophthalmotrope, because then Listing's Law would be violated.

tertiary positions of gaze. Ruete wrote that the ring with screws supporting the model eye represented the 'fat pad behind the eye, the nutshell in which the eye was suspended', quite a modern concept for his time. Donders (1870) later presented his own ophthalmotrope to illustrate Donders' Law. In this model he used gimbal suspension on purpose, to make the pseudotorsion available. This ophthalmotrope was equipped with a camera obscura, to obtain an image of, for instance, the left upper hand corner of the wall in front of us. This image was to be compared with the retinal meridians, which were represented by 4 copper bars surrounding the camera obscura.

The reason for Listing's Law

What is the reason of the existence of Listing's Law or, in other words, why is there a primary position, from which all other eye positions can be reached by simple rotation about a single axis or, in other words, why isn't the primary position in left upper gaze for instance?

Von Helmholtz compared Listing's Law with the minimal energy condition in physics (1863). Applying this principle in a broader sense, one could say that Listing's law is probably the consequence of the fact that the primary position is the average of all eye positions during the day, that most eye movements are directed radially from or to the primary position and that rotations about a single axis are easier to perform than rotation about

100

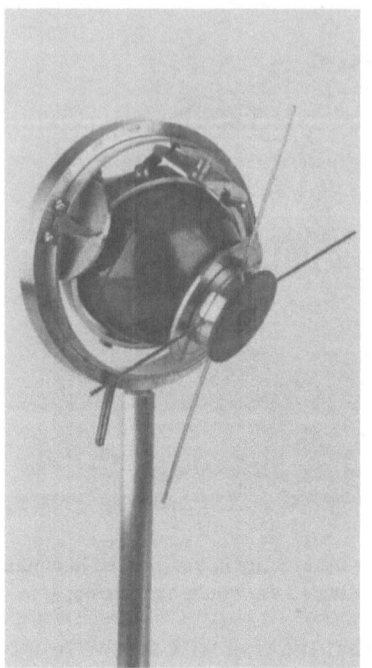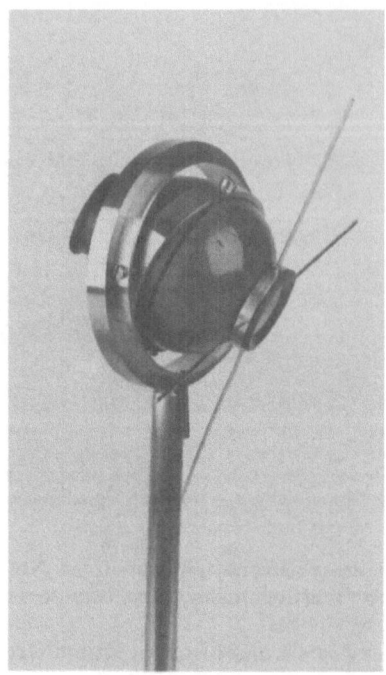

a

Fig. 3a and b. Models to demonstrate and to quantify Donders' pseudotorsion, from the museum of the former Royal Netherlands Ophthalmic Hospital in Utrecht. In these models Donders used gimbal suspension on purpose, to make the pseudotorsion visible (gimbal suspension results in globe rotations that do not conform to Listing's Law). The final version (Fig. 3b) was described by Donders in 1870. The ophthalmotropes were equipped with a camera obscura, to obtain an image of, for instance, the left upper hand corner of the wall in front of us; this image was to be compared with the retinal meridians, which were represented by 4 copper bars surrounding the camera obscura (2 are broken off). The eye rotated in the

two axes or about an axis that changes during the movement. Eye movements from tertiary positions to other tertiary positions do occur, but are less frequent and do not occur predominantly in down-, up-, right- or left-gaze. During eye movement from one tertiary to another tertiary position, Listing's law is fulfilled only if the rotation takes place about an axis that is tilted to Listing's plane by half the angle between the momentary tertiary position and primary position (von Helmholtz 1863): hence an axis that can change during the movement.

The primary position (Ruete 1853), as determined with afterimages (Hering, 1868, p. 74–83) varies over time (von Helmholtz 1910; Schubert 1927), is in down-gaze for convergence (Donders 1876 see below) and varies with head position (Fisher 1922).

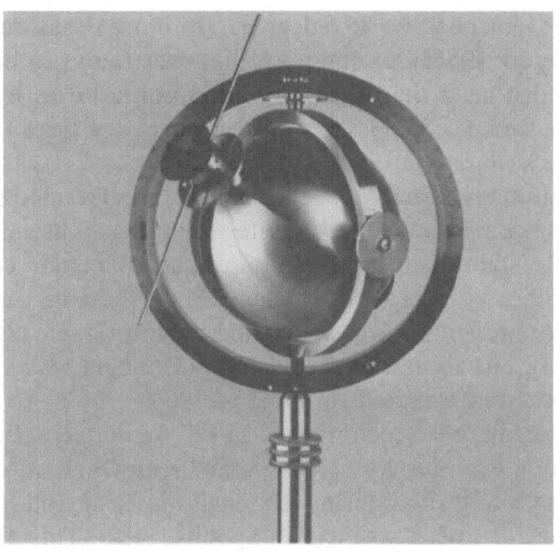

b

inner ring, and the inner ring rotated in the outer ring of the gimbal suspension, the primary and secondary axes of rotation being perpendicular. The outer ring is in Listing's frontoparallel plane and it could rotate in its sleeve-like circular holder, so that the primary axis of rotation could tilt within Listing's plane. Hence, a tertiary position of gaze could be, incorrectly, reached by rotation about the primary horizontal and secondary vertical axes (resulting in pseudotorsion) or by tilting the primary axis of rotation in Listing's plane and subsequent rotation about the primary axis only (in compliance with Listing's Law).

Ocular counterrolling

Donders initially assumed that all rotation of the eyes about the optic axis, was pseudotorsion. The existence of true rotation about the optic axis, 'ocular counterrolling', was denied by him. Ocular counterrolling is a small counterrolling movement of both eyes about the visual axis when the head is tilted towards either shoulder, caused by the otolith reflex. True ocular counterrolling had already been described in 1786 by John Hunter, but had subsequently been overestimated by Hueck (1838), who thought that it fully compensated for up to 28.25 degrees of head-tilt to either shoulder. Actually, Hueck had only seen, not measured, the torsional nystagmus when tilting the head of another person from shoulder to shoulder. Then he measured, in an anatomical study, the distance that the superior oblique tendon could be pulled out of the trochlea, which was 5.5″. He erroneously assumed that the superior oblique muscle had torsional action, exclusively, and given the diameter of the eye he estimated the maximum amplitude of torsional eye movement to be 56.5 degrees. (In more recent measurements, the actual amplitude of ocular counterrolling was found to be 5.64 ± s.d. 2.57 deg on 50 deg head-tilt either way in 55 normal eyes by Nelson and Cope (1971), we found 5.53 ± s.d. 1.95 deg on 45 deg head-tilt either way in 32 normal eyes (Simonsz 1984).

Ruete and Volkmann initially believed Hueck (von Graefe 1854), but later denied the existence of true ocular counterrolling when pseudotorsion was first described by Donders, and the amplitude of ocular counterrolling claimed by Hueck was not found. Hence, Donders' denial of the existence of true ocular counterrolling was supported by von Graefe (1854) and von Helmholtz (1863), but all had to revoke later (Donders 1875), when ocular counterrolling was rediscovered by Javal in 1866.

Ocular counterrolling is accomplished by the concerted action of vertical rectus and oblique eye muscles. The superior rectus and superior oblique muscles of one eye, and the inferior rectus and inferior oblique muscles of the other eye contract, whereas their antagonists relax. This differential use of eye muscles, depending on head-tilt to either shoulder, has important consequences for patients with a palsy of the trochlear nerve that innervates the superior oblique eye muscle.

A patient with a trochlear nerve palsy will prefer a head tilt that confers ocular counterrolling such that the paretic muscle is not needed. Under these circumstances the angle of squint is small and double vision is absent. On head tilt towards the contralateral shoulder the angle of squint gets very large. This principle has been formulated by Nagel (1871), first applied clinically by Baumeister (1874), and elaborated by Hoffmann and Bielschowsky (1900). (Baumeister was a lesser known pupil of Donders; in the same article, however, he also described the dependence of latent nystagmus upon the direction of gaze for the first time!)

Excyclotropia on convergence

A third kind of torsion that has confused investigators is excyclotropia on convergence. Excyclotropia (vertical retina meridians tilting clockwise in the right eye and anti-clockwise in the left eye as seen from the patient's side) on convergence was found by Hering (1868), Donders (1876), Landolt (1876), Allen (1954) and others. We also found it to occur during voluntary convergence using a double-looped scleral search coil (Simonsz and Zee, unpublished results). Why should excyclotropia occur during convergence? The most likely reason was formulated by Donders (1876): Convergence occurs during near vision and near vision is done mostly in down-gaze. If the primary position for near vision is in down-gaze (for the same reason as why

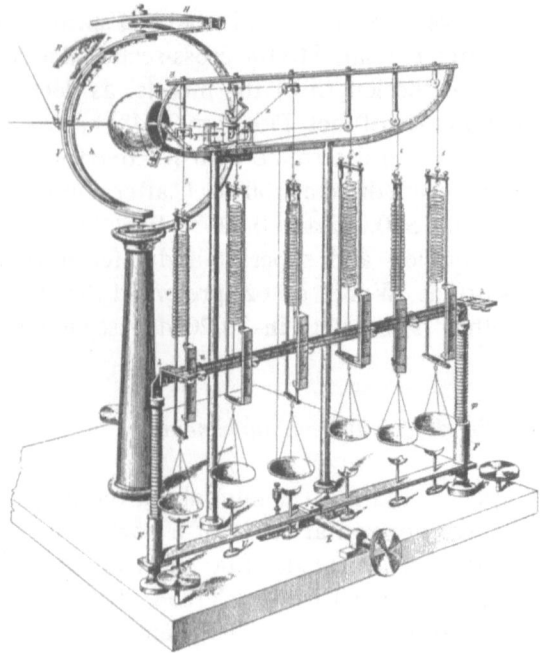

Fig. 4. Wundt's ophthalmotrope (1862). Muscle forces were represented by weights and springs.

the primary position for far gaze is approximately ahead, as discussed above) excyclotropia will occur when converging from gaze ahead. One can calculate and extrapolate the primary position for near vision from the excyclotropia that occurs during convergence from gaze ahead.

Only when converging the eyes by more than 10 deg, corresponding to a target distance of less than 35 cm, excess excyclotropia has been found to occur, not accounted for by assuming a lower primary position for down-gaze, but more than 10 degrees of convergence is of course a very unnatural condition.

Wundt's ophthalmotrope

The most sophisticated model of the nineteenth century was, no doubt, that made by Wundt in Heidelberg, 'ein künstliches Augenmuskelsystem zur Untersuchung der Bewegungsgesetze des menschlichen Auges im gesunden und kranken Zustande' (1862).

Whereas Ruete's model used anatomical variables only, Wundt's model also used physiological variables as muscle forces, represented by springs

and weights. Remarkable in his analysis is that the spring constants of his model muscles were directly related to the cross-sectional area of the muscle and inversely related to the length of the muscle, as determined in post-mortem studies. As a matter of fact, Donders (1848) had already measured the weights of the muscles to determine their relative force. (He found for human eye muscles that were dried at 100 deg C after removal of the tendon: 0.072, 0.0725, 0.0603, 0.075, 0.032 and 0.0265 g for lateral, medial, superior and inferior rectus muscles, and superior and inferior oblique muscles, respectively.) In his article, Wundt (1862) presented the changes of muscle length, force and other parameters in 20/20 deg secondary and tertiary positions of gaze.

Coordinate systems for describing eye movements

In the coordinate system used most commonly in the diagnosis and treatment of squint, first the horizontal angle of a particular gaze position is described, and then the vertical angle (Fig. 5a-b, middle-left). This coordinate system was first employed by Fick (1854). It is an isoazimuth and isolatitude system, similar to the coordinate system used to designate a place on earth and similar to the system used in the Major Amblyoscope and Synoptometer. Its great disadvantage is that, in tertiary positions of gaze, an angle designated, for instance, '30 degrees' is larger vertically than horizontally. (For comparison: on earth the distance between one of the latitude circles and the equator is the same everywhere, whereas the distance between the vertical meridians decreases towards the poles).

Imagine that the coordinate system used to describe eye positions is drawn onto a globe. The observer is in the center of the globe. Imagine that the observer is looking from the center of the globe onto some point on the equator of the globe, and designate this point the primary position. Although the angles of the intersections of the latitude circles and the vertical meridians are all perceived by the observer as rectangular, the directions of the latitude circles and the vertical meridians will, nevertheless, not coincide with the horizontal and vertical meridians of the retina of the observer, they will both be tilted (Donders' law, 1846). If this coordinate system (Fig. 5a, middle left) were projected onto a screen in front of the observer, it would consist of vertical lines (projections of meridians) and horizontal hyperbolas (projections of latitude circles) (Fig. 5b, middle left).

The problems described above would be solved by using a polar coordinate system (Fig. 5a-b, middle right). Here, one angle defines the direction of eye movement and a second angle defines the amount of eye movement out of the primary position, following Listing's Law (Ruete 1853), that 'all

secondary and tertiary positions of gaze can be reached by rotation about a single axis that is perpendicular both to the primary-position gaze direction and to the new gaze direction. However, the trigonometric calculations get very complex when one uses this system and angles of squint would have to be expressed in a totally different way.

Von Helmholtz (1863, 1910) also used a isolatitude-isoazimuth coordinate system, but used isolatitude horizontally and isoazimuth vertically (Fig. 5, top left), the reverse of Fick's system. (An equivalent of this coordinate system on earth would be to have the northpole in Columbia and the southpole in Indonesia.) He argued that the trigoniometric calculations were simpler using this system, when shifts in the reference point, the primary position, occurred: The primary position (Ruete 1853), as determined with afterimages (Hering, 1868, p. 74–83) varies over time (von Helmholtz 1910; Schubert 1927), is in down-gaze for convergence (Donders 1876) and varies with head position (Fisher 1922).

The angles between the horizontal meridians and vertical latitude circles in the system of von Helmholtz are also perceived as rectangular by the observer at the center of the globe but, again, the directions of the horizontal and vertical lines do not coincide, in tertiary positions of gaze, with the horizontal or vertical meridian of the retina of the observer: They are now both tilted the other way.

In a coordinate system that is isoazimuth both ways (meridians both horizontally and vertically on the globe or, projected onto a screen, straight horizontal and vertical lines), the angles between the horizontal and vertical lines are perceived by the observer as larger than 90 deg (Fig. 5a-b, bottom left). An example of the use of this coordinate system is the 'Tangenskala', a frontoparallel screen with straight horizontal and vertical lines on it, introduced by Harms (1941).

Hess (1916) introduced a coordinate system with isolatitude horizontally and vertically (Fig. 5a-b, top right) that became very popular as the 'Hess screen'. It is often used for measurements of the angle of squint in cases of eye muscle palsy. However, the angles between the horizontal and vertical lines of the Hess screen are perceived by the observer as smaller than 90 deg. Kolling and Simonsz (1986) assumed that between the two latter coordinate systems there should be another where all angles would be perceived by the observer as rectangular.

They then re-invented a system based on 'direction circles' (Fig. 5a-b, bottom right). The 'direction circles' represent the direction of the horizontal and vertical meridians of the retina in tertiary positions of gaze (von Helmholtz 1910). When an observer moves his eyes, from some tertiary position, constantly in the direction of the retinal horizontal or vertical meridian, the axis of rotation is neither in Listing's plane (isolatitude), nor

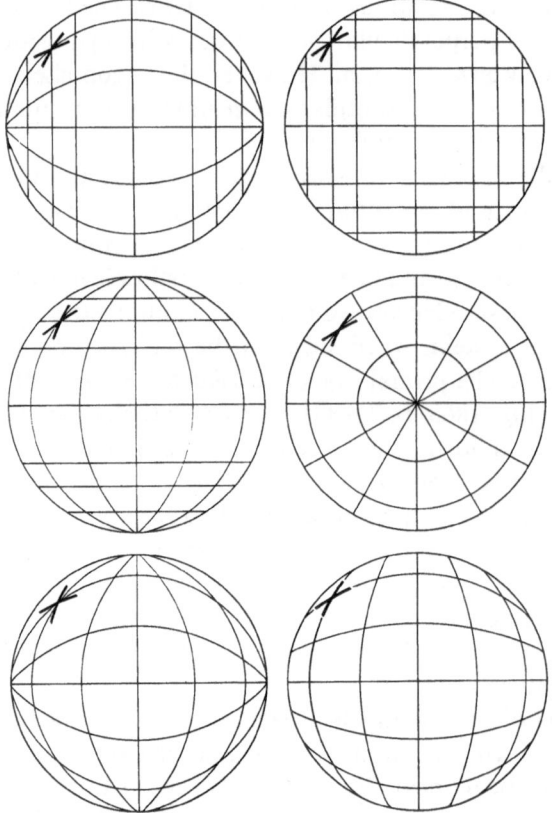

Fig. 5a.

is the axis of rotation perpendicular to the direction of gaze (isoazimuth). The axis of rotation is between these two (Fig. 6). Such an axis is the only possible single axis that the eye can rotate about, going from one tertiary position to another tertiary position and complying with Listing's Law. Now a curious mathematical peculiarity of direction circles is that all direction circles go through the 'occipital point' (von Helmholtz 1910). The occipital point is a point behind the observer. The occipital point is exactly in the direction opposite to the primary position.

Now, for construction of the coordinate system, consider only those direction circles that have either a common horizontal or a common vertical tangent in the occipital point. A series of vertical circles and a series of horizontal circles result (Fig. 7). The direction circles will represent the direction of the horizontal and vertical meridians of the retina in tertiary

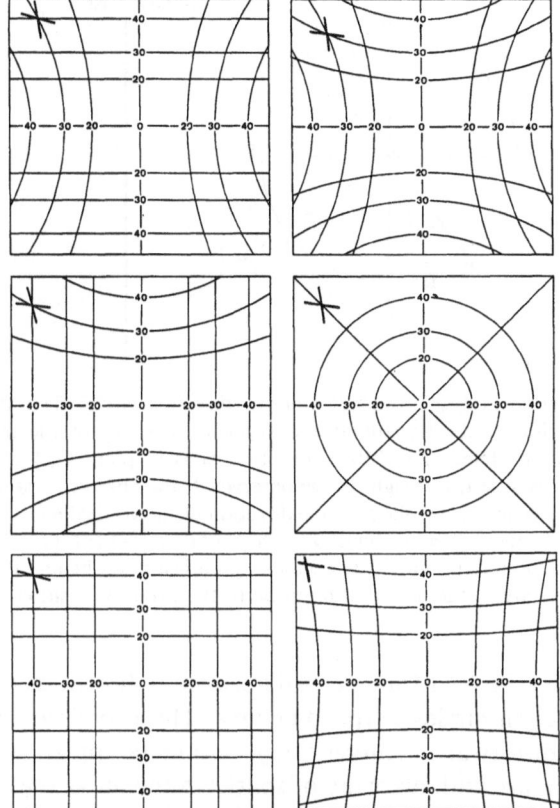

Fig. 5b.

Fig. 5a and b. The six coordinate systems describing eye movements, depicted on a globe (a) and their projections on a frontoparallel screen (b). The observer is at the center of the globe. In each figure, the direction of the horizontal and vertical meridian of the retina is represented by a bold cross. Upper left: the system used by von Helmholtz (1863, 1910) in his eye-movement calculations: isolatitude horizontally and isoazimuth vertically. Middle left: the system used by Fick (1854), isoazimuth horizontally and isolatitude vertically, the coordinate system used on earth, in the Synoptometer and in the Major Amblyoscope. Lower left: the system used by Harms (1941), isoazimuth both horizontally and vertically. Upper right: the systems used by Hess (1916), isolatitude both horizontally and vertically. Middle right: the polar coordinate system. Lower right: the coordinate system proposed by Kolling and Simonsz to be used in strabismus diagnostics, based on the 'direction circles'. The 'direction circles' represent the direction of the horizontal and vertical meridians of the retina in tertiary positions of gaze (von Helmholtz, 1910). Note that the horizontal and vertical meridians of the retina (cross) deviate from the horizontal and vertical lines in all coordinate systems (Donders' Law), except in the direction-circle coordinate system. The direction-circle coordinate system is preferable to the other systems because (1) the direction of the lines represent true horizontal and vertical in tertiary positions of gaze, (2) all intersections are perceived by the observer as rectangular, (3) it is free of Listing's pseudotorsion and (4) the artefact vertical or horizontal deviations that occur using the Major Amblyoscope or Synoptometer, when there is a large horizontal and vertical angle of squint, are avoided.

108

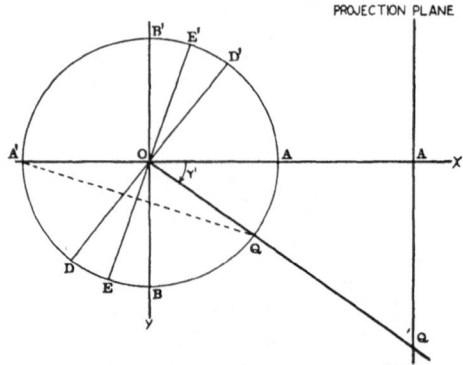

Fig. 6. Axis of rotation in eye movement along a 'direction circle'. The 'direction circles' represent the direction of the horizontal and vertical meridians of the retina in tertiary positions of gaze (von Helmholtz 1910). The observer is at point O, looking in primary position at point A. B' is left, B is right of the observer. If the observer first looks at point Q and then shifts his gaze upwards following the direction of the vertical meridian of his retina, his eyes do not rotate about B'B or about D'D, they rotate about E'E (von Helmholtz 1863, appendix). A' is the 'occipital point'. The occipital point is a point behind the observer. The occipital point is exactly in the direction opposite to the primary position. From Southall, 1937.

positions of gaze (Fig. 8). Moreover, all horizontal direction circles intersect all vertical direction circles perpendicularly. The proof of this (Fig. 9) is relatively straightforward. Interestingly, Donders' pupil Küster (1876) showed, using an arc with an array of sparks in the dark, that the direction circles are perceived as straight lines. This is probably caused by the fact that the horizontal and vertical direction circles intersect perpendicularly, and that they always conform to the horizontal and vertical meridian of the retina: if a line is horizontal everywhere in space, the brain apparently interprets the line to be straight. In the experiments of Küster, a meridian arc (that is projected onto the retina as a straight line) was perceived as curved in tertiary positions of gaze! A more or less similar experiment was done a century later by Nakayama and Balliet (1977): they found that a test-stripe presented in tertiary positions of gaze was set 'vertical' in the dark according to the direction of the direction circles. The perception of the angles of the intersections of horizontal and vertical direction circles being perpendicular is not a 'perceptual illusion' as Held (1970) believed; it really is true! For clinical use as coordinates, the circles can be projected on a frontoparallel screen as hyperbolas having half the curvature of those of the Hess screen.

The direction-circle coordinate system is preferable to the other systems because (1) the direction of the lines represent true horizontal and vertical

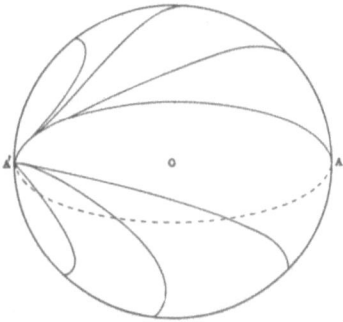

Fig. 7. A family of direction circles. The observer is at point O, looking in primary position at point A. All direction circles go through the occipital point A′. The occipital point is a point behind the observer. The occipital point is exactly in the direction opposite to the primary position. Here, one series of direction circles is shown with a common tangent through the occipital point. The coordinate system proposed by Kolling and Simonsz, based on the direction circles, consists of projections on a screen of a series of horizontal and a series of vertical direction circles. From Southall (1937).

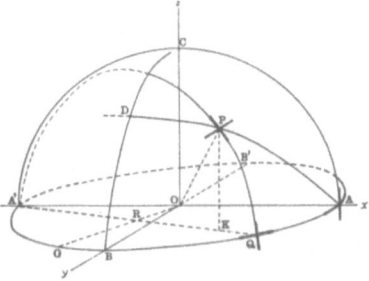

Fig. 8. 3-D drawing of the eye movement described in Fig. 6. A is primary position, A′ is the occipital point and O is the observer. When the observer shifts his gaze from Q to P following the vertical meridian of his retina, the path followed will be a direction circle with OG as axis of rotation. The horizontal and vertical retinal meridians are represented by the cross. Note that the direction of the cross follows that of the direction circle: no pseudotorsion occurs.

in tertiary positions of gaze, (2) all intersections are perceived by the observer as rectangular, (3) it is free of Listing's pseudotorsion and (4) the artefact vertical or horizontal deviations that occur using the Major Amblyoscope or Synoptometer, when there is a large horizontal and vertical angle of squint, are avoided.

Note added in proof

Tweed et al. (1990) have recently published an excellent account on the use of quaternions in describing eye rotation, to get rid of pseudotorsion. There are interesting parallels between the direction circles and quaternions that will need more study.

110

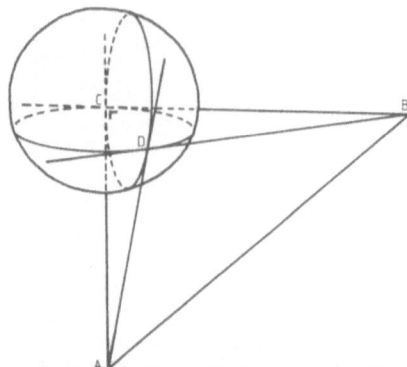

Fig. 9. Proof that all direction circles intersect perpendicularly. Point C is the occipital point. If the circles intersect perpendicularly at C, they also intersect perpendicularly at D, because triangle ABC and ABD are congruent (3 equal sides).

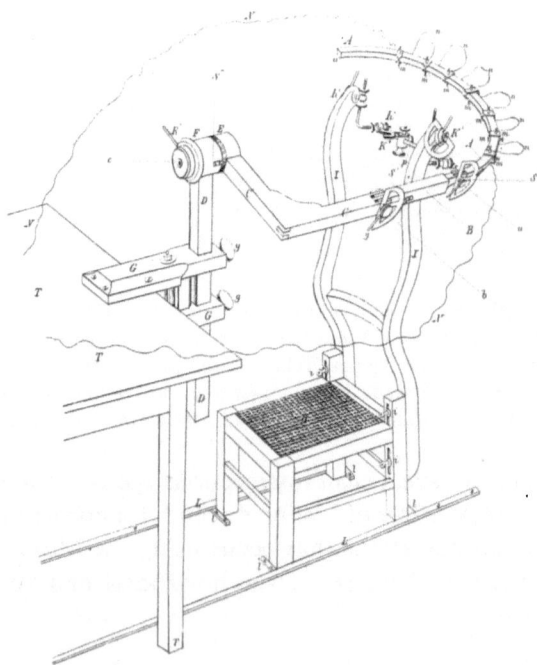

Fig. 10. The observer in Küster's experiments (1876) looked in the dark at an array of sparks (m), on an arc that could tilt like a meridian arc at hinge a, but also like a direction circle at hinge b. The observer sat on the chair 'the wrong way around', his head being fixed with biteboard K. A meridian arc (that is projected onto the retina as a straight line) was perceived as curved outwards in tertiary positions of gaze, a direction circle was perceived as straight!

Acknowledgements

This work was supported by a fellowship of the Royal Netherlands Academy of Arts and Sciences (Dr Simonsz). We wish to thank Dr G. Dagnelie for providing the proof presented in Fig. 9.

References

Baumeister E. Klinische mededeelingen. III. Invloed van de houding van het hoofd bij de gezichtsscherpte bij nystagmus. Jaarlijksch verslag betrekkelijk de verpleging en het onderwijs in het Nederlandsch Gasthuis voor Ooglijders, 15, wetenschappelijke bijbladen (Fifteenth yearly report concerning nursing and education in the Netherlands Ophthalmic Hospital, Scientific suppl.), ed.: Donders FC. Van de Weijer, Utrecht, 1874; 71–73.

Baumeister E. Klinische mededeelingen. IV. Bijdrage tot de diagnose der trochlearisverlamming. Jaarlijksch verslag betrekkelijk de verpleging en het onderwijs in het Nederlandsch Gasthuis voor Ooglijders, 15, wetenschappelijke bijbladen, ed.: Donders FC. Van de Weijer, Utrecht, 1874; 73–76.

Donders FC, Physiologische en pathologische aanteekeningen van gemengden aard, IV: De beweegingen van het menselijk oog. Ned Lancet 1846; 2: 104–158.

Donders FC. Beiträge zur Lehre von den Bewegungen des menschlichen Auges. Holländische Beiträge Anat Physiol Wiss, 1848; 1: 105–45.

Donders FC, Doijer D. De ligging van het draaipunt van het oog. Jaarlijksch verslag betrekkelijk de verpleging en het onderwijs in het Nederlandsch Gasthuis voor Ooglijders, 3, wetenschappelijke bijbladen, ed.: Donders FC. Van de Weijer, Utrecht, 1862; 210–28.

Donders FC. Die Bewegungen des Auges, veranschaulicht durch das Phaenophthalmotrop. Arch f Ophthalmol 1870; 16(1): 154–75.

Donders FC. Über das Gesetz der Lage der Netzhaut in Beziehung zu der der Blickebene. Arch f Ophthalmol 1875; 21: 125–30.

Donders FC. Versuch einer genetischen Erklärung der Augenbewegungen. Pflügers Arch Physiol 1876; 13: 373–421.

Fick A. Die Bewegungen des menschlichen Auges. Zeitschr f rat Med 1854; 4: 101–28.

Fisher MH. Beiträge und kritische Studien zur Heterophoriefrage auf Grund systematischer Untersuchungen. Alb v Graefes Arch f Ophthalmol 1922; 108: 251–84.

Harms H. Über die Untersuchung von Augenmuskellähmungen. Graefes Arch Ophthalmol 1941; 144: 129–49.

Held R. Two modes of processing spatially distributed visual stimulation. In: The neurosciences, second study program, ed: Schmitt FO. Rockefeller University Press, New York, 1979; 317–24.

von Helmholtz H. Über die normalen Bewegungen des menschlichen Auges. Graefes Arch Ophthalmol 1863; 9(2): 153–214.

von Helmholtz H. Handbuch der Physiologischen Optik, Vol 3. 3rd ed, Leopold Voss, Hamburg & Leipzig, 1910.

Hering E. Die Lehre vom binocularen Sehen. Wissenschaftliche Abhandlungen, Band 2. Engelmann, Leipzig, 1868.

Hess WR. Ein einefaches messendes Verfahren für Motilitätsprüfung der Augen. Zeitschr f Augenheilk 1916; 35: 201–19.

Hoffmann FB, Bielschowsky A. Die Verwerthung der Kopfneigung zur Diagnostik von Augenmuskellähmungen aus der Heber- und Senkergruppe. Alb v Graefes Arch f Ophth 1900; 51: 174–185.

112

Hueck. Die Achsendrehung des Auges. Dorpat, 1838.

Hunter J. The use of the oblique muscles. In: Observations on certain parts of the animal oeconomy. London, 1786.

Kolling GH, Simonsz HJ, van Dijk B. Die Bedeutung des Koordinatensystems für die Motilitätsdiagnostik. In: Augenbewegung und visuelle Wahrnehmung, Proc 1st Symp Bielschowsky- Gesellschaft f Schielforschung, ed: Mühlendyck H, Göttingen, October 1986. Enke Verlag, Stuttgart, 1989.

Küster F. Die Direktionskreise des Blickfeldes. Arch f Ophthalmol 1876; 22(1): 149-210.

Listing JB. Beitrag zur physiologischen Optik. Göttinger Studien. Göttingen, Vandenhoeck and Ruprecht, 1845.

Nagel A. Über das Vorkommen von wahren Rollungen des Auges um die Gesichtslinie. Alb v Graefes Arch f Ophth 1871; 17: 237-64.

Nakayama K, Bailliet R. Listing's Law, eye position sense, and perception of the vertical. Vision Res 1977; 17: 453-57.

Ruete CGT. Das Ophthalmotrop, dessen Bau und Gebrauch. Göttinger Studien. Göttingen, Vandenhoeck und Ruprecht, 1845.

Ruete CGT. Lehrbuch der Ophthalmologie. Braunschweig, 1846; 2nd edition, Vol. 1, 1853; 36-37.

Ruete CGT. Leerboek der Ophthalmologie, in het Nederduitsch bewerkt en van aanteekeningen voorzien door dr. Donders, off. v. gen. der tweede klasse bij 's Rijks kweekschool voor militaire geneeskundigen. Utrecht, C. v.d. Post Jr, Amsterdam, C.G. v.d. Post, 1846.

Ruete CGT. Ein neues Ophthalmotrop, zur Erläuterung der Functionen der Muskeln und brechenden Medien des Menschlichen Auges. Leipzig, Teubner, 1857.

Schubert G. Studien über das Listingsche Bewegungsgesetz am Auge. I. Mitteilung. Pflügers Arch Physiol 1924; 205: 637-68.

Schubert G. Studien über das Listingsche Bewegungsgesetz am Auge. II. Mitteilung. Pflügers Arch Physiol 1927; 215: 553-87.

Simonsz HJ. Investigations of ocular counterrolling and Bielschowsky head-tilt test, stiffness in passive ocular rolling and displacement of recti eye muscles. PhD Thesis, University of Amsterdam, 1984.

Simonsz HJ. The mechanics of squint surgery: Length-tension measurements of human eye muscles, their implementation in a computerized model, and analysis of squint surgery with the model. Habilitionsschrift (thesis) University of Giessen, to appear in Acta Strabologica C.E.R.E.S.(Dr J.B. Weiss), Paris, 1990.

Southall JPC. Introduction to physiological optics. Dover Publications, New York, 1937.

Tweed D, Cadera W, Vilis T. Computing three-dimensional eye position quaternions and eye velocity from search coil signals. Vision Res 1990; 30: 97-110.

Tweed D, Vilis T. Geometric relations of eye position and velocity vectors during saccades. Vision Res 1990; 30: 11-127.

Volkmann AW. Über die Mechanika der Augenmuskeln. Ber Verh Sachs Wsch 1869; 21: 28-69.

Wundt W. Ueber die Bewegung der Augen. Arch f Ophthalmol 1862; 8(2): 1-87.

Wundt W. Beschreibung eines künstlichen Augenmuskelsystems zur Untersuchung der Bewegungsgesetze des menschlichen Auges im gesunden und kranken Zustande. Alb v Graefes Arch Ophthalmol 1862; 8(2): 88-114.

Address for correspondence: H.J.Simonsz, Netherlands Ophthalmic Research Institute, P.O. Box 12141, 1100 AC Amsterdam, The Netherlands.

Documenta Ophthalmologica **74**: 113–118, 1990.

Ocular manifestations during the French travels of discovery to Australia from Lapérouse (1741–1788) to Dumont D'Urville (1790–1842)

PIERRE AMALRIC
6, rue St. Clair, 81000 Albi, France

I had the honour and the privilege to go to Sydney in February 1988 with a Minister of the French Government for the inauguration of the Lapérouse Museum in Botany Bay. You may know that, on the first days of the Australian continent, a French navigator, Lapérouse, arrived at the same time as Commodore Phillip with his convicts. The memory of Lapérouse is still very vivid in Australia as it is in mine, particularly in my home town, Albi, where he was born in 1741. His statue stands on one of the main squares of the town.

I have chosen this subject to pay hommage to the Australian nation which he was one of the first to visit, and to pay hommage to the Academia Ophthalmologica Internationalis because, when we study the history of Australia, we are struck by the number of countries which have participated in its discovery, its creation and its expansion.

The name Australia, which is often incorrectly attributed to its geographical position, is in fact due to the Spanish navigator Mandena, who wanted to honour the great duke of Austria, Charles V's brother who was particularly esteemed by the Spanish and the Flemish.

During the following century, the Portuguese made a lot of discoveries and they probably initiated the maps illustrating the first geographical representation of this continent which was unknown until then. These maps were drawn in France, at Dieppe, and later in England at the court of King Henry VIII. However, they remained ignored in both these countries until the end of the XVIIIth century and during this long lapse of time, in the XVIIth century, Holland, which became the great rival of Portugal on the seas, gave to this country the name of 'New Holland'. All this shows that, prior to the immortal discoveries of James Cook and of the English navigators of the XVIIIth century, long pages of history had been drawn.

The XVIIIth century was a period of exploration of the last unknown continents and England was particularly outstanding because of the quality of its sailors and of their discoveries. France, the rival of England for more than 60 years, sent important expeditions over the seas and some navigators made significant discoveries in the scientific field.[1]

The Scotsman James Lind made a comprehensive study on the action of lemon juice as a preventive or curative treatment of scurvy. His book was even translated shortly after its publication. However, the English admiralty ordered the application of this treatment among sailors only one year after Lind's death and we had to wait for more than eighty years before the French followed the same example. Some said that if lemon juice had been adopted earlier, American Independence would have been more difficult to achieve. However, a humorist said that we owe to lemon juice Napoleon's ultimate defeat.

From Bougainville to Lapérouse, numerous advances had been made and Cook's precepts were carefully followed by the French.

The anti-scurvy action of malt was not proven but the conservation of the fermented vegetables in barrels enabled the preservation of anti-scorbutic substances. We know that the rat, who makes a perfect synthesis of ascorbic acid, constituted an excellent means to prevent the disease in these sailors. Unfortunately, scurvy remained the main cause of mortality in European fleets. Moreover, dysentery was frequent and Cook lost more than 40 men in some days. By alcalinization of the medium, dysentery provoked an important vitamin deficiency in the affected sailors.

The clinical history of these sailors was impressive; they presented an excessive vascular fragility associated with diverse infectious manifestations. Hemorrhages often occurred in any point of the organism, more particularly in mucous tissues.

Ocular manifestations were considered as epiphenomenons when compared with the gravity of their general condition of health. As concerns Lapérouse's expedition, both surgeons on board, Rollin and Lavaux, managed to maintain perfect sanitary conditions, and this was a real progress as it appears from studies of medical ship's papers carried out by Professor Kerneis from Nantes. More than two hundred theses, based on official documents dating from that period, have been published in Nantes. They give us perfect information concerning the observations of the surgeons of the French expeditions in the Pacific and Oceania.[2]

During Lapérouse's expedition, Rollin carried out the first studies of

[1] In spite of all these rivalries, English and French scientists established close links. The relationships between both countries were never interrupted and such famous men as Banks and Buffon, Priestly and Lavoisier, were associated in a common research for progress.
[2] Recently, a Franco-Australian expedition has discovered bones of the sailors of Lapérouse's expedition, shipwrecked in Vanikoro. None of these bones reveals signs of scurvy.

anthropology performed in United States and Kamtchatka. He probably continued his research in Australia but the last part of his report disappeared in the Vanikoro's shipwreck. He had to treat several patients presenting serious injuries and he even trepanned his colleague Lavaux who had been injured by the natives.

The chaplain of the expedition, the Father Receveur died after a serious ocular injury. We wonder how such a wound may provoke death by penetration of a foreign body in the orbit. Some, as Doctor Niaussat, have envisaged the hypothesis of cephalic tetanus. Nevertheless, any ocular epidemia or hemeralopic disorders have never been mentioned during the expedition.

If serious ocular infections were frequent on the voyages from Africa, they were almost inexistent during the great voyages through the Pacific and yet conditions of hygiene were extremely precarious.

Trachoma was brought from Egypt by the English and Napoleonic armies.[3] It spread to America via slave-ships but it is odd to notice that English convicts did not bring the disease to Australia.

At the end of the XVIIIth century, marked in 1788 by the taking up of New South Wales by Commodore Phillip's squadron, Dr. White performed medical investigations and created in Sydney the first hospital of this continent.

Some time later, Bonaparte sent Baudin's expedition to Australia to inspect the coasts. From a medical point of view, it was a real disaster. The commander, unaware of the need to stop at ports of call, remained at sea for periods over 100 days. In fact, it has been experimentally demonstrated that it is necessary to board every sixty days in order to get vegetable products which are rich in vitamins. This rule had been strictly applied by Cook and Lapérouse, but not by Baudin whose sailors were exhausted when they arrived in Sydney where they had to stay for a long time before they recovered.

The following voyages had less serious medical implications since they benefited from the revolutionary advances made in the field of nutrition. James Lind's works are particularly important as well as Lazzaro Spallanzani's studies showing that spontaneous generation did not exist and that the preservation of vegetables by heat could be beneficial. This discovery was at the origin of the booklet edited by Nicolas Appert on canned food. This principle was applied to the English navy and even to the French navy in spite of the Continental System.

---

[3] See Wagemans, M. and Bijsterveld, O.P., 'The French Egyptian campaign and its effect on ophthalmology'. Docum. Ophthalmol. vol. 68 Nos 1, 2, pp 135–144 (1988).

In fact, the high death-rate of sailors in the XVIIIth century decreased progressively as general medical disorders were amended. It is only from that period that ocular manifestations began to be reported.

As you may know, the term 'hemeralopia' which has been misused since the time of Hippocrates, is still incorrectly applied. We know that it referred to a retinal deficit provoking disorders of night-vision or night-blindness. In the first treatises of ophthalmology, its treatment consisted in the absorption of animal liver.

The chemical nature of vitamin-deficiency was described much later by Fuson and Christ (1936). We know that vitamin A is derived from carotenoids which are converted into vitamin A by the intestine and mainly stocked by the liver. The anomaly induces the deficiency which appears only after a 60 days period of deprivation; it results in night-blindness and keratinization of epithelial tissues of the body. This has been experimentally demonstrated.

But these facts, which were unknown in the XIXth century, are not the only ones explaining the visual disorders observed in the sailors at that period. Numerous theses, inspired by Dean Kerneis of Nantes or published in other countries, report that hemeralopia is often associated with scurvy either before or after its onset. We know that it is an 'infectious' disease affecting crews or entire companies of soldiers. It may be observed in any part of the world but it has mainly been reported in the tropics. A distinction must be made between hereditary hemeralopia which is a stage of late pigmentary retinitis, and accidental hemeralopia which results from a dietetic dysfunction.

If we stick to the problem of hemeralopia in the French navigators of the Pacific, we can see that this disorder is noted in every log-book. Beyond the myths which characterize the life of sailors, today we can say that the surgeons on board made an objective study. To define the stage of hemeralopia, the authors relied on the patients' ability to discern stars of first, second or third order, or a candle-light in the night which was progressively moved away. Comparison was made with a normal subject and the seriousness of the disorder depended on the distance.

We also know that the colour of the eye could play a role and some theses report cases with blond-haired and blue-eyed subjects.

Finally, beyond the conditions of diet and fatigue which contributed to the appearance of the disorder, the notion of sunlight is to be considered. The sun interfered in diverse manners, either by its position in the tropics, by its reflection on the sea, or by its scintillation.

Vitamin deficiency, and conditions of hygiene often hard to maintain, constituted premonitory elements but sun-burns took diverse aspects according to the different cases. Maculopathy was often observed and its manifestations extended from the simple transient amblyopia to the definite burn of cones. Nyctalopia was only clinically described in the treatises published in the beginning of the following century.

As a conclusion, we can say that during these expeditions, sufferings were considerable for these men who sailed for the discovery of new continents and who participated in the creation of Australia.

References

Auffray Y. Thèse no 2834 du 16/6/82 Fac. Med. Nantes, sur le chirurgien navigant Arena Rabel.

Baldy EL. De l'héméralopie épidémique. Thèse Strasbourg 1859.

Bataille A. Le journal médical de Adolphe Pierre Lesson, chirurgien de Dumont D'Urville sur l'Astrolabe. Thèse Med. Nantes 1978.

Bonnafy G. Considération sur l'héméralopie. Thèse Paris 1870.

Boudet. De l'héméralopie en particulier des pays chauds. Thèse Montpellier 1873.

Brossard de M. Influence des contraintes médicales dans les voyages au XVIIIe siècle d'Anson à Lapérouse. Colloque Lapérouse Albi 1985. Ed. Association Lapérouse Albi-France.

Carre A. La santé et les expéditions au XVIIIe siècle. Colloque Lapérouse Albi 1985. Ed. Association Lapérouse Albi – France.

Chaussonet. De l'héméralopie aiguë. Thèse Paris 1870.

Colin. De l'héméralopie et de son traitement. Thèse Paris 1865.

Comme A. Quelques considérations sur l'héméralopie épidémique observée à bord de l'aviso Le Limier pendant la campagne de l'Océan Pacifique en 1876.

Coquerel C. De la cécité nocturne. Thèse Paris 1849.

Dechambre A & Lereboullet L. Dict. Encycl. des Sciences médicales T. 13e, p. 145 (Hem-Her) Paris, 1888.

Dubois E. Héméralopie lors d'un scorbut dans une campagne du Pacifique Thèse Paris 1879.

Duke Elder S. Vit A deficiency – System of Ophthal. Vol. X, p. 496 H. Kimpton 1967.

Fontan J. De l'héméralopie tropicale. Bull. et Mem. Soc. Fr. Ophtalmologie 1884 pages 111–121 et Arch Med. Navale 1884 XLI; 324–29.

Gaziello C. La prophylaxie du scorbut sz Cook à Lapérouse. Albi 1985. Ed. Association Lapérouse Albi-France.

Gourbeil J. Héméralopie endémique; traitement par huile de foie de morue à l'intérieur. Thèse Paris 1864.

Guepratte A. Héméralopie des pays chauds. Observations recueilles à bord de la Frégate l'Armide. Mission de Madagascar 1846. Gaz. Médicale de Montpellier 1847 – VIII, 6.

Guerenne de la C & Kerneis JP. Le voyage autour du monde du pharmacien R.P. Lesson et les essais de la seconde génération des conserves de Nicolas Appert. Bull. de la Soc. Histoire de la Pharmacie. A paraitre.

Guicheteau T. Traitement du scorbut utilisé par Jérôme Bellefin dans l'expédition de Nicolas Baudin. Colloque Lapérouse Albi 1985. Ed. Association Lapérouse Albi-France.

Guicheteau T & Kerneis JP. Etude à travers les chrononavigrammes des responsabilités médicales de Baudin en Australie en 1801–1803. A paraitre. à Canberra à l'occasion du Bicentenaire de l'Australie.

Guillemeau. Tr. des maladies de l'oeil qui sont en nombre de 113. Chapitre X, Paris 1585.

118

Jobet. Thèse Montpellier 1829.

Kerneis JP & Delmas A. A propos d'un manuscrit original concernant l'enseignement de l'anatomie à l'Ecole de Chirurgie de Rochefort, l'enseignement de Jean Cochon Dupuy et de ses successeurs. Colloque Lapérouse Albi 1985. Ed. Asociation Lapérouse Albi-France.

Kerneis JP. Le journal médical manuscrit du 3e chirurgien P.A. Lesson, à Vanikoro avec l'Astrolabe de Dumont d'Urville en 1828. Colloque Lapérouse Albi 1985. Ed. Association Lapérouse Albi-France.

Laveran. Note sur la nature de l'héméralopie. Rec. Mem. de Med. militaire Paris 1858. 2e s XXI 233/238.

Lecaillon P. Nicolas Rollin, chirurgien navigans Lorrain 1778–1787. Thèse de medecine Nantes 1978.

Le Frapper. Thèse Montpellier 1850.

Maitre Jan Traité des maladies de l'oeil, 1707.

Mackenzie W. Practical treatise on the diseases of the eye. 2nd ed. Night blindness. London 1835; 880.

Martialis. De l'héméralopie. Archives Med. navale Paris 1869. Pp 39–49.

Mereau A. De l'héméralopie par cécité nocturne. Thèse Paris 1860.

Mirouze J. Progrès révolutionnaires de la nutrition à l'époque de Lapérouse: les grands navigateurs, premiers bénéficiaires. Colloque Lapérouse Albi 1985, ed. Association Lapérouse Albi-France.

Neboux. Note sur l'épidémie d'héméralopie. Bul. Générale de Thérapeutique Paris 1858 T LV, 461–419.

Nozeran A. Quelques considérations sur l'héméralopie observée à bord de la frégate amirale La Pallas au cours d'une campagne sur l'Océan Pacifique Montpellier Médical 1864 XII; 247–257. Thèse Montpellier 1865.

Ollivier. Thèse Montpellier 1847.

Ouvrard CF. Quelques remarques sur l'héméralopie surveillée à bord du Lavoisier pendant une campagne en Océanie. Thèse Paris 1858.

Pirion. Considération sur l'héméralopie et le scorbut. Arch. Med. navales 1865. IV; 405–424.

Payen CV. Sur l'héméralopie ou cécité nocturne. Thèse Paris 1816.

Quemar C. Considérations sur l'éméralopie. Rapport chirurgien major frégate l'Alceste 1854–1856. Compte rendu soc. Bilogie de Paris 1857. 2e s III. Pp 248–251 et thèse 1858.

Richard H. L'alimentation au cours de l'expédition de d'Entrecasteaux (1791–1794).

Rigaudeau, Privat C. Sur le chirurgien navigans Adolphe Simon Neboox. Thèse no 1989 du 5/5/78 Fac. de Med. de Nantes.

Riviere P. L'héméralopie observée à bord de la canonnière La Cordelière pendant une campagne dans les mers des Indes. Thèse Montpellier 1864.

Sauber PAG. De nyctalopie, Jenae 1693.

Taulier G. L'alimentation des Marins. Thèse Paris 1873.

Tayeau F, Kerneis JP. Les médecins de Lapérouse au cours du grand voyage. 1785–1788.

Warlomont E. Traité pratique des maladies de l'oeil par W. Mackenzie 4e Ed. Cécité nocturne, section XII, p. 733.

Address for correspondence: P. Amalric, 6, rue St. Clair, 81000 Albi, France.

Documenta Ophthalmologica **74**: 119–123, 1990.

The blind Belisar as beggar

WOLFGANG JAEGER
Heidelberg, FRG

Abstract. The blind Belisar as an example of the sudden fall from honour and glory to poverty and distress inspired not only Rembrandt but also several artists from the 17th to the 19th century. The contemporary historians report that Belisar was dismissed by Justinian because of envy and distrust and that he died in poverty. Details about his blinding can be found only in an epic of the 12th century. A report is given about the different gruesome techniques of blinding that existed during the centuries of Byzantine empire.

The name of Belisar reminds us of the period of the emperor Justinian during the Byzantine empire's Golden Age. Works of art dating from this period are still known everywhere and the emperor's codification of Roman Law, the Corpus Iuris Civilis, has had its impact on European civilization for many centuries.

Glory and power of the East Roman empire at that time was mainly due to the victorious battles which the Byzantine army fought under the command of Belisar against Vandals, Goths and Persians. Because of these victories, North Africa, Sardinia and Corsica were re-occupied and after the fall of the Ostrogoth kingdom, Italy again became part of the empire. At Ravenna, which was conquered by Belisar in 540 AD, we can still admire the mosaics of the church of San Vitale, founded after the conquest of the city. They represent Justinian and the empress Theodora, surrounded by their attendants and adorned with all the luxury of the Byzantine court [1]. What a different spectacle is offered by Rembrandt's drawing: 'The blind Belisar as beggar' (Fig. 1). The drawing dates from the late 1650's, when Rembrandt's house and all his possessions had already been put up for public sale and he himself, completely impoverished, was only attended by his faithful maid Hendrijke [2]. Therefore it is comprehensible that he was moved by the fate of Belisar, who at one time was the most famous general of the Byzantine empire and later became a victim of envy and distrust. Emperor Justinian stripped him of all his charges and put him into prison. A year later he was released from imprisonment; he lived in poverty and died after two years. The inscription on Rembrandt's drawing reads as follows: 'erbarmt U over den armen bellisaro die nochtans wel was in groot aensien

120

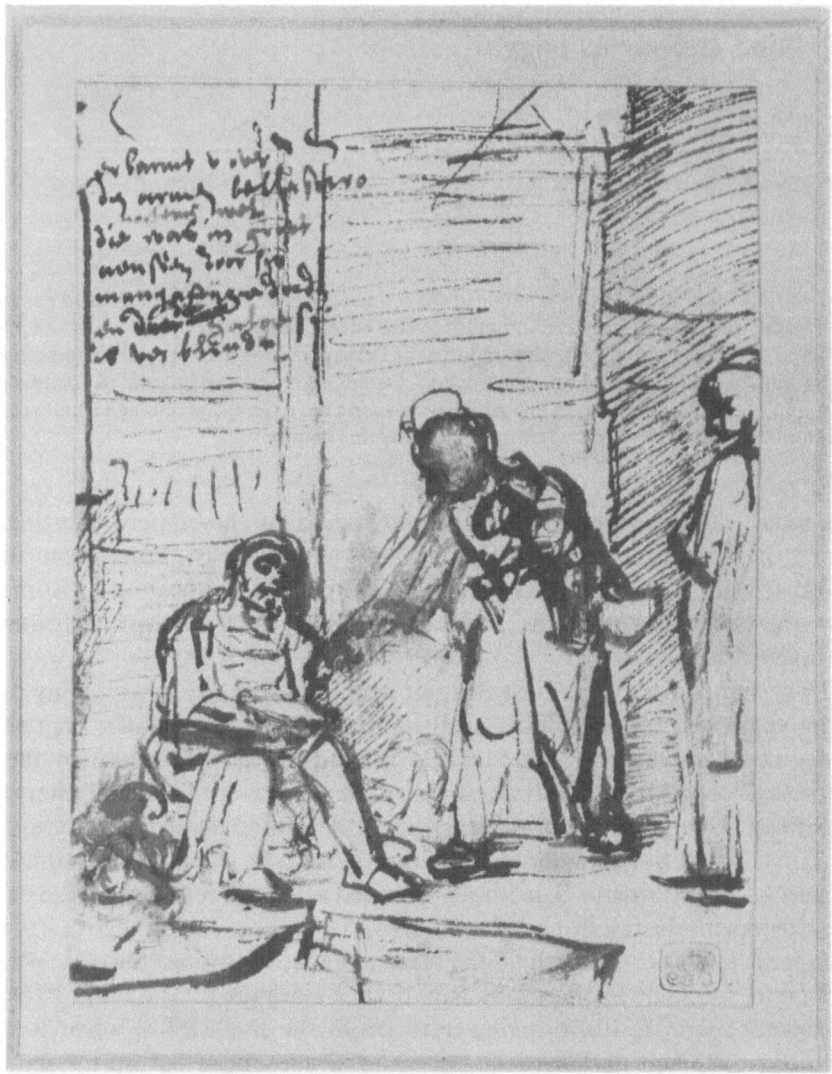

Fig. 1. Rembrandt: The blind Belisar as beggar. Staatl. Museen Berlin. Kupferstichkabinett.

door syn manhaftyge daden en door de jaloesy is verblindt.' 'Have mercy upon the poor Belisar who once was held in great esteem for his gallant deed and who was blinded because of envy.' This example of the sudden fall from honour and glory to poverty and distress, caused by envy and ingratitude rather than mistake or vice, has inspired not only Rembrandt but several artists from the Baroque period to the 19th century [3]. Just a few of the most famous examples: Both a picture and a drawing originate from a contemporary of Rembrandt's in Italy, Salvator Rosa [4]. In the Rococo style, this topic was even for porcelain figures, as shown for instance by figures from Lunéville. An example from the beginning of the 19th century is a picture by Jacques Louis David in the Louvre. At the same time, at the beginning of the 19th century, the character of Belisar drew attention also from dramatic poets as well as from the composers of operas. Shortly before King Otto of Greece landed in Nauplia, during a time of wide-spread Philhellennism in Bavaria, Eduard von Schenck, a minister of King Ludwig I and talented dilettant poet, wrote the tragedy 'Belisar' in the style of Schiller. He dedicated this tragedy to King Ludwig I [5]. Shortly after Donizetti composed the opera 'Belisario'. It originates from the best and most productive period, just immediately following his most famous opera Lucia Lammermoor [6].

In all these pictorial, literary, and musical representations, the blindness of Belisar plays the crucial part – as already written on the inscription of Rembrandt's drawing. According to the legend, Belisar was blinded by order of the emperor so that he would be eliminated as a possible pretender to the throne [7]. Procopius, the most important historian of this time, however, only reports that Belisar was dismissed by the emperor because of envy and distrust and that he died in poverty. Yet, Narses was appointed as his successor, who, being an eunuch, was no possible pretender to the crown. The description of the blinding of Belisar can only be found in an epic of the 12th century derived from earlier sources, as for example a tourist's guide to Constantinople. The unknown author of the epic seems to have freely contaminated the fate of Belisar with that of another general, who was blinded in 866 by order of an envious and suspicious emperor and made a beggar [8]. According to the narrative of the epic Belisar was first blinded by a golden chain or bond which had been put around his head very tightly. Only some time later, because of new accusations and slander of his enemies, the emperor had him blinded in the full sense of the word.

The history of the Byzantine emperors shows a nearly unbroken chain of this gruesome practice, partly even as mass executions [9]. The emperor Basilius II, for example, ordered the blinding of 14,000 Bulgarian prisoners of war and – I cite literally: 'For every 100 men one man was left one eye, so that the whole file of blinded could be lead back to the Bulgarian Tsar.' During such mass blindings the eyes were either cut out or burned by means of glowing steel. A repeated blinding could also be performed by the different techniques that existed in Byzantium [10]. One possibility was not to perforate, but only to roast the cornea, by means of a glowing piece of metal, which was called Mydros. This resembles the treatment of the ulcus serpens with cauterisation before the introduction of sulfonamides and antibiotics. A Byzantine author reports for example that during the blinding of a ten year old child, the eyes were only parched [11]. This was meant as a special privilege, as so-called philantropeia, since the eyes lost vision only gradually by this treatment. According to the extent of the parching of the cornea, a residual vision would be regained. In such a way the blinding could also be dosed that complete blindness occurred only temporarily. This method was being employed when the rival had to be eliminated only for some time, as, for example, during the repeated dynastic quarrels. The rival was mostly a member of the royal family.

A Byzantine specialty which probably was employed in the legendary process of Belisar's blinding was the blinding by means of a glowing basin, which was held in front of the victim's eyes, after his lids had been forcibly fixed in an opened position. The technical term of this process was 'abacinare' (coming from Basinus = Bakynos = basin). This kind of blinding, too, could be repeated and is often testified in the history of Byzantium [12]. After the invention of photocoagulation it was assumed that this 'abacinatio' could well have been a light coagulation of the retina. This assumption for instance seemed to explain the legendary self-blinding of the philosopher Democritus. He is said to have blinded himself by means of a metallic mirror [13]. On a drawing of Salvator Rosa's [14] one can see him with the mirror. Probably the artist supposed that Democritus fixated the sun with the help of this mirror. In this case there would exist some relation to the photocoagulation. But such a technique is not reported in the historical sources. For the abacinatio, however, it is highly unlikely that the low intensity of a glowing basin could have been sufficient for a photocoagulation. Rather one has to assume that the 'abacinatio', too, was performed as a measurable blinding by thermal lesion of the cornea.

The popular epic on the fate of Belisar was written at a time when the empire was torn by internal strife, rivalries, and court intrigues and, therefore, approaching its decline and fall. So the story of Belisar was meant as a warning since it demonstrated how envy, distrust, and civil discord always destroy those members of the community who are able to prevent the final catastrophe. The moral advice to be taken from the history of Belisar and the pity for the man who has fallen from the peak of human fortune led to its popularity in European art and poetry from the 16th to the 19th century.

Acknowledgements

I am thankful for all the information about artistic and historical aspects of this topic I got from Prof J.S. Held (Old Bemington), Prof W. Sumowski (Stuttgart), Prof P.A. Riedl (Heidelberg) and Dr K. Bergdolt (Heidelberg). Most valuable help I received from Prof A. Dihle (Heidelberg), who gave me historical and linguistic comments about the sources of the Byzantine literature and gave me assistance in the English translation of the manuscript.

References

1. Bovini G. & Matt Lv. Ravenna. Du Mont Schauberg, Köln 1971.
2. Held JS. Der blinde Tobias und seine Heilung in Darstellungen Rembrandts. Mit einem Vorwort von W. Jaeger. Die medizinhistorische Bedeutung der Tobiasheilungen Rembrandts. Brausdruck Heidelberg 1980. Belisar Fig. 20.
3. Pigler A. Barockthemen II. Berlin-Budapest 1956. p. 425–426.
4. Mahoney M. The drawings of Salvator Rosa. New York–London 1977 I p. 461–462 and II Fig. 41, 1. – Salerno L. Salvator Rosa. Florence 1963. Fig. 32.
5. Schenck Ev. Belisar. Romantisches Trauerspiel in 5 Aufzügen. Reclam o.J.
6. Ashbrook W. Donizetti and his operas. Cambridge 1982.
7. Beck HG. Geschichte der byzantinischen Volksliteratur. In: Byzantinisches Handbuch im Rahmen des Handbuchs der Altertumswissenschaft II, 3. S. 150–153. C.H. Beck. München 1971.
8. Follieri E. Il poema bizantino del Belisario. In: La poesia epica e la sua formazione. Academia Nationale dei Lincei 1970. Quaderno 139. p. 583–651. (publication in Greek and Italian).
9. Schaab M. Die Blendung als politische Maßnahme im abendländischen Früh- und Hochmittelalter. Diss. Heidelberg 1955. Reporting the practices in the history of the Byzantine Emperors, demonstrated by the Diss. of O. Lampsides Athens 1949.
10. Jaeger W. Die verschiedenen Formen der Blendung und ihre Darstellung in der Kunst. Proceedings XXX. International Congress of the history of medicine. Düsseldorf 1986. Ed. H. Schadewaldt. Vicom K.G. Leverkusen 1988. S. 591–603.
11. Georgios Pachymeres 3, 16.
12. Hoppe U. Ophthalmologische Beiträge zur Technik der Blendung. Diss. Heidelberg 1962.
13. Gellius, Noctes Atticae 10, 17; Plutarch de curiositate 12 p. 521 C/D.
14. Wallace RW. Salvator Rosa's Democritus and L'umana Fragilità. The Art Bulletin 50 (1) 20–26 (1968) Fig. 9.

Address for correspondence: W. Jaeger, Mozartstrasse 17a, 6900 Heidelberg, FRG.

Documenta Ophthalmologica **74**: 125–133, 1990.
© 1990 *Kluwer Academic Publishers.*

Eye references in the Homeric Epics

J. FRONIMOPOULOS & J. LASCARATOS
6 Neofytou Vamva St., 10674 Athens, Greece

Abstract. After a short introduction to the Homeric Epics, the name of Homer and the time and place where the poems were written, the authors refer to the terms of the eyes and to the verses where they are found. Among these terms, the most important is the term οφθαλμός, the first term for the eye in ophthalmology, which has remained throughout the years unchanged.

Finally, they refer to the injuries of the eyes, the participation of the two sons of Asclepios in the Trojan campaign and to the verses including the classical paragraph '. . . a doctor is more capable than the other men . . .'

Both Epics relating to the cardinal human values: prudence, temperance, fortitude and justice, contain the lofty ideal of human excellence, called by the Greeks αρετή .

The Homeric Epics, the *first writing* in Greek history, are the creation of a divine poetic soul, and comprise the most poetic achievements of the human language, intellect, imagination and heart.

According to tradition, a poet by the name of Homer existed in ancient times. Historians like Hirodotus, Thucydides and others, mention that this poet, apart from the 'Odyssey' and the 'Iliad', wrote other marvellous poems which unfortunately have not been preserved.

Concerning the name Homer, scholars could not discover a hellenistic etymology to this name. However, among other historians, Eforos writes that the word Homer derives from two words μή ὁρᾶν , which means 'not see', corresponding to 'blindness' and coinciding with traditional legend, that the poet was blind (Fig. 1). Other investigators considered the name Homer to be a nickname, and Welcker thought that the name derives from two Greek words ὁμοῦ ἀίρειν , which means together join, because the poet composed his epics by joining together small poems.

Probably, the name Homer comes originally from the area of Asia Minor. By 1950, most scholars in England and the United States came to the agreement that the structural and artistic finish of the epics require us to assume the existence of a single poet, the traditional Homer.

The poet is assumed to have worked with a technique of oral composition, and made use of traditional saga material, and earlier epics, parts of which may derive from the late Mycenean age. The historical element of the saga has, of course, been overlaid by myth, legend and folk tale.

126

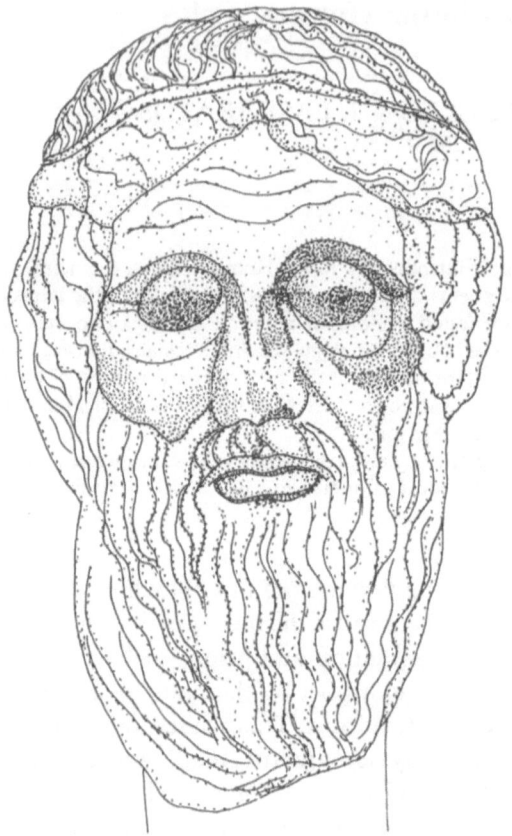

Fig. 1. Homeros (München, Glypothek).

Writing was known in Greece during the eighth and seventh centuries B.C., and the Homeric Epics, originally small and of different form, were later joined together, revised, corrected and written in the sixth century B.C. Thus the final text acquired today's form.

The place where the Epics were written originally, is the Aegean Sea, along the coast of Asia Minor.

The 'Iliad', the earlier of the two epics, related the adventures of the Greeks at the siege of Troy, is arranged around a central unifying theme of the wrath of Achilles and its disastrous consequences for both Greeks and Trojans.

The 'Odyssey' tells of the homecoming of Odysseus, his travels and adventures on the way, and the vengeance which he took on the base suitors of his wife, Penelope, when he reached his home, Ithaca.

Both epics, apart from their literary value, contain important references to eyes. These references are considered to be the first in ophthalmology, some of them remaining unchanged to our days.

Let us begin with the description of Athena's eyes. Homer uses the word γλανκῶπις meaning 'bright blue eyes', which is repeated in many verses, as in the verse IL Δ 439, 'ωρσε δέ τούς "Αρης, τούς δέ γλανκῶπις Αθήνη. . .', (. . . some were aroused by Aris and others by the bright blue eyed Athena . . .), and in many other verses.

Poetic expression is given also to Hera's eyes, with the word βοῶπιζ, which means 'wide oxlike eyes', eyes like those of a cow, ox or bull, as in the verse IL Δ 50, '. . . τόν δ ημείβετ᾽έπειτα βοῶπις ποτνία ερη. . .' (. . . the venerable wide-eyed Hera responded. . .).

Also the term ἐλίκωψ, used with the meaning brilliant, lighting eyes, round shaped eyes. It is mentioned in the verse IL Π 569, '. . . Ωσαν δέ πρότεροι Τρῶες ἐλίκωπας᾽ Αῶααούγ. . .' (Trojans were the first to push back the Achaians with round-shaped eyes). Homer uses the following anatomical terms for the external parts of the eyes:

1. βλέφαρα , a word meaning 'eye lids'.
   It is mentioned in the verses IL T 15, 16, 17, 'ἐν δέ 'οσσε δεινόν υπό βλεφάρων εἰ σέλαζ ἐξεφάανθεν. . .' (. . . and his eyes flashed strongly under his eyelids like fire . . .).

2. ὀφρύες-ἐπισκήνιου both terms having the meaning 'eyebrows' as in the verses OD I 389, '. . . πάντα δέ οἱ βλεφάρ᾽ ἀμφί καί ὀφρύας ἔνσεν αὐτμή. . .', (. . . and all around the eye lids and the eyebrows), IL P 136 '. . .πᾶν δέ τ᾽ἐπισκ-ήνιου κάτω ἔλκεται ᾽όσσε καλύπτων. . .'(and with frowning eyebrows, covers his eyes. . .).

3. ῥίσαι , a term probably used for the optic nerve. It is mentioned in the verse OD I 390, '. . . σφαραΥεῦτο δέ οἱ πυρί ῥίσαι. . .' (. . . and crackling in the fire the roots (the optic nerves) of his eye. . .).

4. Θέμελα, a term used for the 'orbit'. It is mentioned in the verse IL Ξ 493, '. . . τόυ τοθ ὑπ ὀφρύος οὔτα κατ ὀφθ αλμοῖο θέμελοι. . .' (. . . now, he wounded him under his eyebrow, in the orbit. . .).

Homer also uses the following terms for the globe of the eye (bulbus oculi)

1. ὀφθαλμός , a term which means 'eye'. It is mentioned in many verses, as in IL E 290, 291 '. . . βέλος δίθινεύ Αθηνη ρίνα παρ ὀφθαλμόν, λευκος δ ἐπέρησεν ὀδόντας. . .' (. . . Athena aimed the arrow towards the nose, near the eye and pierced the white teeth. . .).

2. ὄσσε , term meaning also 'eyes', mentioned in the verse IL Δ 431, 'τόν δέ σκότοβ κάλυψεν...' (... and his eyes were covered by darkness...).

3. ὄμματα , again, a term meaning 'eyes', mentioned in the verse IL Γ 397, '...στήθεα θ.' ἱμερόευτα καί'ὄμματα...' (... her desirable breasts and her flashing eyes...). The term ὄμματα is also used metaphorically, meaning 'glance', 'gaze', 'look'. It is mentioned in the verse IL Γ 217, '... στάσκευ ὑπάι δέ ἴδεσκε καί χθονός ὄμματα πήζας...' (... he was standing and looking downwards, having his glance fixed on the ground...).

4. ὦπα (ωψ), a term also used with the meaning 'eyes'. It is mentioned in the verse IL I 372, '... ουδ αυ ἐμοιγε τετλαίη κύνεος πέρ ἐάν εἰς ὦπα ἰδέσθαι...' (... and he didn't dare look in my eyes, even though he is as fierce as a dog...). The word (ὦπα metaphorically means 'appearance', 'glance'. It is mentioned in the verse OD X 405, '... δεινός δ εἰς ὦπα εἰδέσθαι...' (... his appearance seems terrifying...).

5. Υλήυη , term which means 'eye', 'the lightening of the eye'. It is mentioned in many verses, among them, OD I 390, '... Υλήνης καιομένης...', (... the eye which was burning...).

6. φάος-φάεα , meaning 'eye' and also 'lucid', 'the sparkling light of the eye', 'light of the eyes'. It is mentioned in many verses, among them in the verse IL Φ 415, '... Ωs ἄρα φωνήσασα πάλιν τρέπειν ὄσσε φαεινω...' (... as he said these words, his lucid eyes turned elsewhere...). The word φάος , metaphorically means feeling of joy, happiness, safety, victory. It is mentioned with this meaning in the verse IL Π 15, '... κύσσε δέ μιυ κεφαλήν τε καί ἄμφω φάεα καλά...' (... and full of happiness he was kissing his head and his sweet eyes...).

7. ὀπωπή , term with the meaning 'appearance of the eyes'. It is mentioned in the verse OD Γ 97, '...ἀλλ εύ μοι κατάλεζον ὅπως ηυτνσας ὀπωπῆς...' (... and tell me exactly what you saw with your eyes...). The work ἠπωπή metaphorically means 'sense of vision', as in the verse OD I 512, '... χειρῶν ἐζ'οδυσῆος ἀμαρτησεσθαι 'οπωπης...' (... I will lose my vision by Odysseus' hand).

8. ἄχος means 'sorrow', 'grief', 'pain', as expressed by the eyes. It is mentioned in the verse IL Y 282 '...κάδ ἄχος οί χύτο μύριον ὀφθαλμοῖσι...' (... and endless sorrow flowed in his eyes...).

9. δακρυόφι , word meaning 'shedding of tears after sorrow, joy, grief, mourning', mentioned in many verses, such as OD Y 704, 705, '... τω δε οι ὄσσε δακρυόφι πλήσθεν...' (... her eyes were full of tears...), and IL P 695, '...τώ δέ οί ὄσσε δακρυόφι...' (... his eyes were shedding tears...).

In some verses of the Epics, we meet description of the primitive knowledge of the sense of vision, which according to the theory of the ancient Greeks, about concepts of light and vision, was:

Light comes out of the brain and is projected like a flash, via the eyes, to objects to be seen. This theory was developed later by the Epicurean philosophers.

It is mentioned in the verse IL Δ 150, '... ὀφθαλμῶν τε βολαί...' (... and the lighting from his eyes...). It is also referred to in the verses describing the sparkling eyes of Achilles, full of wrath against the Trojans, for the killing of his friend Patrocles. IL T 365, 366, '... τὼ δ ὄσσε λαμπέθην ὡς εἴ τε πυρός σέλας...' (... and his eyes flashed with a fiery gleam...), also in the verses referring to Hector, who was full of anger, during the battle, with eyes shooting fire, IL M 466, '... πυρὶ δ ὄσσε δεδήει...' (... fire was coming out of his eyes...).

Homer uses the following terms for the various visual disorders:

αμαύρωσις , meaning 'diminishing vision',
δυσκορασία , meaning 'obscurity',
ἀχλύς , meaning 'dimness', 'cloudiness',
σκότος , meaning 'dark', 'obscure', 'death',
νύκτα , meaning 'night', 'death'.

The term αχλύς is mentioned in many verses, amon them in IL O 668, '... τοῖσι δ ἀπ ὀφθαλμῶν νεφος ἀχλύας ὦσεν Ἀθηνη.....' (... and Athena took from their eyes cloudiness and mist...). Also in the verse IL Π 344, where the term αχλύς has the meaning of dimness by fainting; '...κατά δ ὀφθαλμῶν κέχυτ ἀχλύς...' (... his eyes grew dimn...). The terms σκότος (dark), νύκτα (night), ἀχλύς (dimness), associated with the word 'eyes', have the meaning of death, as in the verses IL Δ 525, 526, '... εἰ δ ἄρα πᾶσαι χύντο χαμαί χολάδες, τόν δέ σκότος κάλυψε...' (... and all his entrails were poured out and his eyes covered the dark (meaning that he died)... ; IL E 310 '... ἀμφί δέ ὄσσε κελαινη νύξ ἐκάλυψε...' (... and both his eyes covered the black night...(he died); IL O 578, '... τόν δέ σκότος κάλυψεν...' (and his eyes covered the dark (death).

παράβλωπες is another term used by Homer with the meaning 'squint', as in the verse IL I 503, '... καί γάρ τε Λιταί εἰσί Διός κούραι μεγά-λοιο, χωλαίτε ῥυσαί τε παράβλωπες † ὀφθαλμῶν...' (... because and Lites, are daughters of the great Zeus, lame, wrinkled, and with squinting eyes...).

Homer uses the term κυνζω which is a verb, which the meaning 'to make leprous', and metaphorically, 'to dazzle', or 'to make dim or opaque', 'give a disgraceful appearance', 'ugly', 'humble'. It is mentioned in the verses where Athena, touching Ulysses' eyes with her magic wand, makes him ugly, with a disgraceful appearance. OD N 429, '... Ὡς ἄρα μιν φαμένη ῥάβδω ἐπεμπάσσατ Ἀθήνη... (433) κυνζώσω δέ οἱ ὄσσε παρος περικαλλέ ἐουτι (402) ὡς ἀυ ἀεικάειος πᾶσι μνηστήρσι φανίετις...' (... thus Athena said, and touched him with a stick... and his eyes, which before were sparkling, became dim,.. so that he would present a disgraceful appearance to the suitors...).

Homer describes the movement of the eyes and uses the term παπταίων for the rotation of the eyes, as in the verse IL P 673, '... Ὡς ἄρα φωνήσας ἀπέβη ζανθὸζ Μενέλαος πάντοτε παπταίων ὡς † ἀϊτιός...' (... thus he spoke and left the blond Menelaos, rolling his eyes in all directions like an eagle...). This term is also used in other verses.

The poet also describes eye injuries, all quite serious, including injuries to neighbouring areas of the skull, those being fatal. They are mentioned in many verses, among them in IL N 615-619, '... ὁ δὲ προσιόντα μέτωπον ρινός ὕπερ πυμάτης λάκε δ ὀστεά τώ δέ οἱ ὄσσε παρ ποσίν αἱματόεντα χαμαί πεσόυ ἐν κουίησιν ἰδυώθη δέ πεσών...' (... just as he was coming against him, hit him at the base of his nose, and the bones were broken, and his two blood-filled eyes fell down in the dust at his feet, and he dropped down dead.).

In the verses IL Π 345-350, there is an injury mentioned with bleeding in the eyes, probably hyphaema or hyposphagma, '... Ἰδομενεύς δ Ερύμαντα κατά στόμα νηλέϊ χαλκῶ νυξε τό δ ἀντικρύ δόρυ χαλκέον ἐξεπέρησε νέρθευ ὑπ ἐγκεφάλοιο, κέασσε δ ἄρ ὀστέα λευκά. Ἐκ δέ τίναχθεν ὀδόντες, ἐνέπλησθεν δέ οἱ ἀμφω ἀίματος ὀφθαλμοί τό δ ἀνά στόμα καί κατά ρίνας πρῆσε χανών...' (... Idomeneas hit Erymanta in the mouth with the pitiless weapon; the spear made of copper went through to the other side, beneath the brain and broke the white bones, filling his eyes with blood, which bubbled up through his open mouth and nostrils...).

Traumatic enucleation is referred to in an injury during a battle when Pinelaos, sovereign of Biotia, hit Ilionea's forehead with a spear just beneath the eyebrow, resulting in excision of the eye-globe, and the spear remained in the orbit. IL Ξ 493, '... τόν τοθ ὑπ ὀφρύος οὖτα κατ ὀφθαλμοίο θέμελα ἐκ δ ὦσε γλήνην...' (... now he wounded him beneath the eyebrow in the root of his eye, resulting in its excision...).

Homer also cites wounds causing blindness by burning. It is mentioned in the verse referring to the burning of the Cyclops's eye by Ulysses, with a pole heated in the fire. OD I 387-390, '... Ὡς τοῦ ἐν ὀφθαλμῶ πυρίηκεα μοχλόν ἐλόντες δινεόμεν, τόν δ αἱμα περίρρεε θερμόν ἰόντα. Πάντα δέ οἱ βλέφαρ ἀμφί καί ὀφρύας εὑσεύ αὐτμή, γλήψης καιομένης σφαραγεύντο δέ οἱ πυρί ρίζαι...' (... Thus, we turned the heated pole in the eye of Cyclops, and as it was hot and stuck in the eye, blood moistened his face around the eye, eyebrows and eyelashes were toasted by the fire and burned the globe and the roots of his eye were sizzling in the fire... (Fig. 2).

Homer mentions blindness as a punishment in the verse IL Z 138-139, '... Γῶ μέν επειτ ὀδύσαντο θεοί ρεία ζωόντες ...καί μέν τυφλόν Κρόνου πάϊς...' (...Gods who live without any effort and Kronos' son, blinded him...). Also in the verse IL T 91-92, '...πρέσβα Διόζ θυγάτηρ"Ατη, ἡ πάντας ἀᾶται,

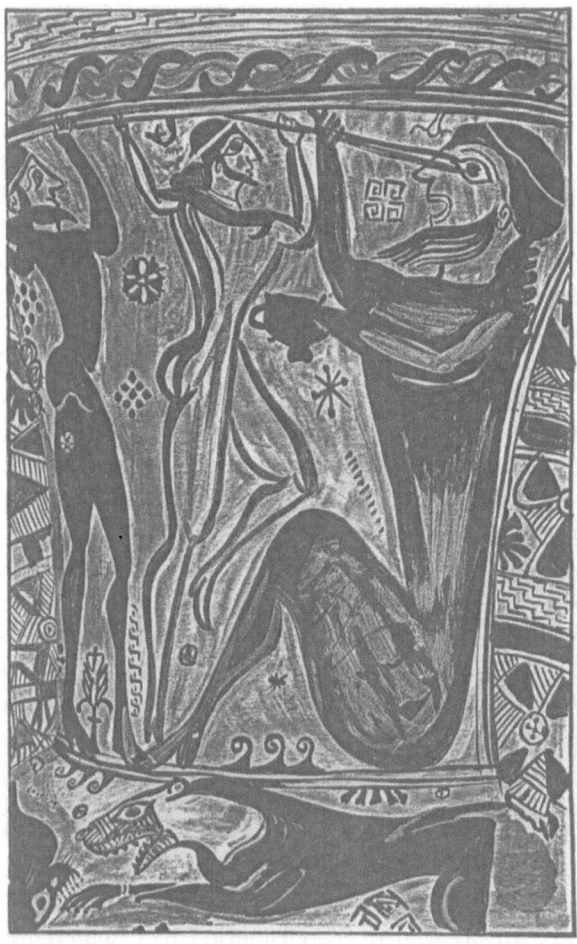

Fig. 2. The Cyclops Polyphemos holdine the crater of wine, tries to remove the burning pok from his eye.

Before ending, I would like to mention the two sons of Asclepios, Machaon and Podalirios, who participated in the Trojan campaign, not only as doctors, to treat the wounded warriors, but also to participate in the war as commanders of the army from Triki, Ithomi and Ichalia. It is mentioned in the verse IL B 732–733,... τῶ αὖθ' ἡγείσθην Ἀσκληπιοῦ δύο παῖδε ἰητῆρ ἀγαθῶ, Ποδαλείριος ἠδέ Μαχάων...' (.... they had as commanders the sons of Asclepios, capable doctors, Podalirios and Machaon...).

Medicine was also performed by the heroes, like Achilles, Menelaos, Diomidis, Nestor, Ulysses and other, who participated in the Trojan war; they were taught medicine by the Centaur Cheiron who lived in the Pilion mountains.

The Epics include the most ancient manifestations of medicine wrought by faith and experience. Described in the Epics are 140 injuries with an estimated mortality of 77.6%, primitive surgical treatments and use of remedies. But with all these human aids, there is the divine refuge in magic, which continued to play an important role in the ancient Greek medicine for many centuries. Thus human weakness seeks refuge in the Gods, appealing to them for salvation. An interesting remark on war injuries is that the painters who painted warriors and battles on vases and amphoras, rarely illustrated wounded warriors with serious and fatal wounds, thus avoiding ugly and unaesthetic pictures, and were restricted to presenting the fighters, the winners and the heroes in all their magnificence and dignity. In the verses referring to the above-mentioned sons of Asclepios the two doctors, we meet the paragraph 'doctor is more capable than other men', which remained classic to the present day. The phrase is included in the verse IL Λ 510, '...
αὐτίκα δ Ιδομενεας προσεφώνησε Νέστορα δῖου. 'ὦ Νέστορ Νηληϊάδη, μέγα κῦδος Αχαιῶν, ἀργει, σῶν ὀχέων ἐπιβήσεο, παρ δέ Μαχάων βαινέτω ἐς υἦας δέ τάχιστ᾽ἔχε μώνυχας᾽ἵππους.ἰητρός γάρ ἀνήρ πολλών ἀντάξιος᾽ἄλλων. ἰούς τ ἐκτάμνιεν ἐπί τ᾽ἤπια φάρμακα πάσσειν...᾽, (... immediately Idomeneas called the divine Nestor, Nestor, son of Nilea, great glory of Achaians, forward, step in your carriage, take besides you Machaon, and guide your horses as fast as you can to the ships because a doctor is more valuable than other men, capable of removing arrows and placing on the wounds fine powder of soothing herbs).

Conclusion

In conclusion, we can say that in the Homeric Epics, which give an elegant and gracefully poetic narration of the complete geography, history and civilisation, mainly of the pre-Hellenic period, we found interesting terms on eyes. Among a number of them, the most important is the term ὀφθαλμός (ophthalmos), the first term for the eye in ophthalmology, which has existed throughout the years unchanged. Both Epics, 'Iliad' and 'Odessey', illustrate the cardinal human values: prudence, temperance, fortitude and justice, which correspond to the duties of man towards himself and to others, and are distinguished by the human sense of value and dignity of man. Thus the Epics concerning the lofty ideal of human excellence, called by the Greeks 'arete' (αρετή) came to be the the prized possession of Greek literature.

References

1. Bernardakis N.D. Three lessons on Homer's Epics. Ed. Pandora, pp. 370–373, 1865.
2. Croiset, Alfred and Maurice. The history of the Ancient Greek Literature. Transl. into Greek by A. I. Pournaras, V. A., Athens, 1938.
3. Encyclopedia Americana. Vol. XIII, p. 4182, 1963.
4. History of Greek Literature. Hadas, Moses, New York, 1950.
5. Kallitsounakis, J. Article on the Homer. The Great Greek Encyclopedia. V. 18, p. 864–876 (contains the most important bibliography).
6. Leirpfeld, D. Treatises on Home. Published in "Kathimerini", 20 and 27 March, 1939. Leirpfeld, D. The Homer's Epics. Published in 'University of Kathimerini', V. A, p. 14–22 and V.B, p. 94–95, 1934.
7. Mistriotis, G. The history of the Homers' Epics. Leipzig, 1867. Edition in Greek, Athens, 1903.
8. Murray, G. The history of the Ancient Greek Literature, Trans. into Greek by S. Menandros, Athens, 1922.
9. Sideris, Z. Odyssey and Ilias. The Library of the Ancient Greek Writers. Ed. J. Zacharopoulos, Athens, 1939.
10. Schoemann, G.F. The Homer's Greece. Ed. 1861, Trans. into Greek by G.F. Tzerepi, Athens, 1867.
11. Vlachos, A. Homer's Topic. Athens, 1886.

Address for offprints: J. Fronimopoulos, 6 Neofytou Vamva St., 10674 Athens, Greece.

Documenta Ophthalmologica 74: 135–139, 1990.

Eye votives in the Asklepieion of ancient Corinth

S. CHAVIARA-KARAHALIOU
Krokida 44, Kiaton, Greece

Abstract. The present study describes the eye votives that were found in Asklepieion of ancient Corinth during the excavation by the American School of Classical Studies and attempts to diagnose the possible diseases.

Comparable to the widespread fame and reputation of ancient Corinth was the fame of her Asklepieion, or hospital, as we would say today.

Asklepieia were establishments with impressive architecture. They had dormitories for the patients, special areas for the various cures that were performed, a recreation hall, dining hall, baths, a sanctuary where visitors would sacrifice the animals offered to Asklepios and special areas where the sacred animals (snakes, dogs and cocks) were kept, as well as storerooms for food and other materials.

In the *Korinthiaka* of Pausanias there is a very brief mention of the temple of Asklepios 'near the exit from the city'.

Beyond the theater lies the gymnasium, and not very far from it are two temples, one dedicated to Zeus, the other to Asklepios. Close by is the spring Lerna which is well described by Pausanias: 'Columns stand around it, and benches have been constructed to refresh those who have entered in the summertime. Next to this gymnasium are two temples, the one of Zeus, the other of Asklepios. The images of Asklepios and Hygeria are of white stone, but that of Zeus is of bronze'. (Paus. 2.4.5).

In this remote time, illness and its development, identified as they were with the divine, could only inspire the sick with feelings of fear, reverence and thankfulness. These feelings they would try to express with their gifts to the gods, with hymns, prayers and votives – the so-called 'models' (τύπια) – which exist even in our day as symbols and tokens of the gratitude of the sick who having become well with divine help, usually dedicate representations of the afflicted member of the body.

In the ancient Asklepieia there were many such models fastened to the walls in such a way as to suggest to the ill visitor the power of the healing god on the one hand, and on the other to proclaim the skill of the healer-priests of the temple: a manner, in short, of professional advertisement.

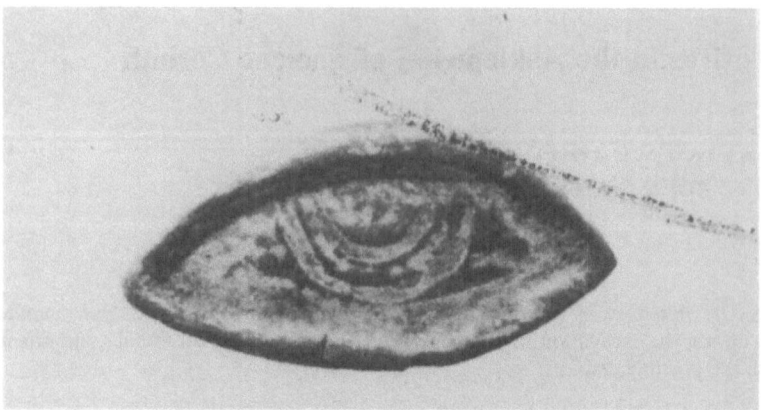

Fig. 1. Votive representing a deep scalding of the eyeball.

These models, ancient writers inform us, were of precious metals – gold or silver – if dedicated by a wealthy person, or of bronze and other less costly metals or alloys if the dedicant was less wealthy. For the poor the simple solution was to use clay.

In the excavations of the Asklepieion of ancient Corinth conducted by the American School of Classical Studies, they found a great wealth of votives, almost exclusively of clay, various metal tools and vessels which were used for the preparation of various medications.

In these healing-shrines, in addition to the various diets, gymnastic exercises, massages and baths, certain operations were also performed as is proved by the various implements which were discovered in the excavations. Besides the lancing of abscesses, stitching of wounds and setting of fractures, they also performed more serious operations on the inner organs such as the stomach and uterus, etc.

The votives which were found in the excavations, apart from their artistic merit, have for us physicians perhaps a greater significance because they provide evidence for the anatomical, physiological and surgical knowledge of the physicians of the Asklepieia of that distant epoch.

From the great amount of votives chiefly of the upper and lower extremities we can conclude that in the healing-shrine of ancient Corinth, 'the Asklepiads had special abilities in orthopedics.' Likewise, votives of ears confirm that otology belonged to the curative skills of the establishment.

The small number of eye-votives found in the excavations is striking in comparison with the votives of other parts of the body. The amount is relatively small also when compared with the number of patients and diseases of the organ of sight. For example, in the inscriptions from the

137

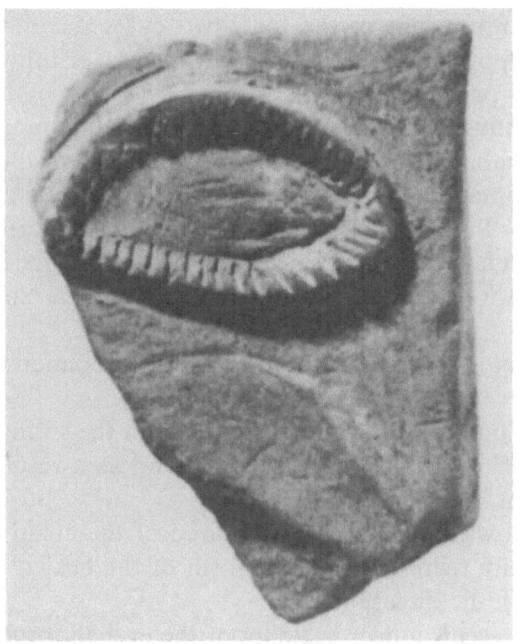

Fig. 2. Normal eyeball with ectropion of the lower lid.

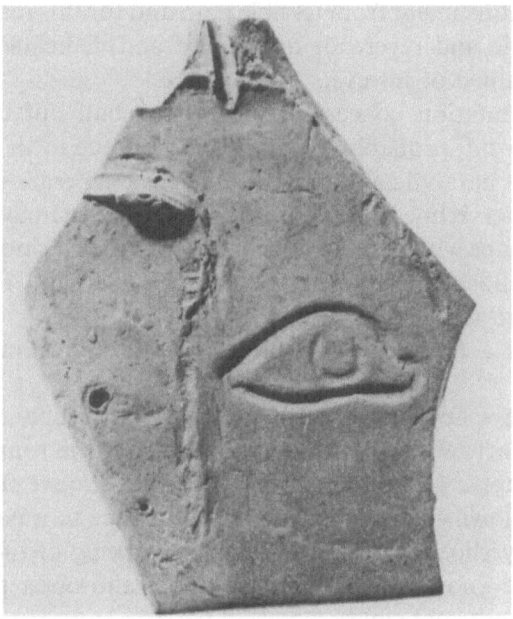

Fig. 3. The votive is a fragment of a longer plaque.

Asklepieion at Epidauros eight of the forty-two cures mentioned are of diseases of the eye – approximately one-fifth – while at Corinth we have an overwhelmingly small percentage.

We all know that injuries to the eyes are very common among farming people as were the inhabitants of the area at that time. But also the various inflammations and contagious diseases such as trachoma must have been everyday occurrences. Purulent dacryocystitis, sties, and abscesses of the eyelids must have been fairly frequent since even today, in a time of plentiful antibiotic eye-washes, these are fairly frequent complaints among rural populations.

The small number of eye-votives discovered is in our opinion due to two responses:
1) their small size resulted in their being easily lost in the silting-up which occurred here both with the passage of time and as a result of earthquakes in the area;
2) the specialized knowledge which was required of the creative artist in order to successfully represent the final form of the healed eye, or the change wrought by the disease itself.

The first votive represents a deep scalding of the eyeball, probably from lime, which has destroyed its entire surface and resulted in total ectropion. Despite the fact that the eye is functionally useless, perhaps the patient found relief at the establishment from terrible pain and for this reason he felt that he owed gratitude and reverence to the god and dedicated to him a likeness of what remained of his eye.

The second representation concerns a normal eyeball but there is an ectropion of the lower lid, probably a senile ectropion due to the advanced age of the patient or a paralytic ectropion caused by a general neurological illness. Apparently dacryrrhoea, which is agonizing, led the patient to the Asklepieion, and perhaps with some simple operation (the closing of the gap between the two eyelids with stitches) he found relief, and for this he dedicated the model to the god.

The third votive is a fragment of a larger plaque and admits of two interpretations.
1) The well-formed eye appears to be a right eye with a fine and correct portrayal of the narrow, angular outer canthus and the rounded inner canthus. On the upper left there appears clearly a groove from which fluid evidently is flowing. Probably this is a reference to a pathological condition of dacryrrhoea, caused by the over-working of the lacrymal gland which as we know is located in the upper and outer part of the eye-socket in the lacrymal cavity.
2) The outer interpretation is that maintained by the American School of

Classical Studies that conducted the excavations: that it represented the eighth cure recorded on the inscriptions of the Asklepieion at Epidauros.

As Aravantinos explains it, a one-eyed suppliant lost his sight and sought the help of Asklepios. During his incubation in the shrine he dreamed that the god visited him and poured a healing eye-wash into his eye. In the morning he left the establishment with sight in both eyes.

We can accept this view if we believe that on the left side of the plaque the eyelids are barely indicated and from above the drug is being poured from a special vessel, while on the right side there was a healthy eye exactly as this naive patient believed to have happened with his imaginary eye. If the plaque had been preserved entirely, the interpretation probably would be easier. The explanation of Aravantinos of this cure is that at some point inflammation had closed the eyelid of the healthy eye and when the eye-wash was applied and the patient awoke, he saw again but he thought that he was seeing with both eyes.

The priests encouraged this exaggeration because they were very well aware of the power of psychotherapy through exaggeration, the autosuggestion of hallucinations and the faith in the power of the god. Part of the therapy in the Asklepieia was the effect on the psyche of the patients caused by the sight of the many votives which were exhibited 'in a conspicuous place.' The majority of these had great artistic merit as well.

References

1. Ἀποστολάκι Γ. Ἀνατομική τοῦ ανθρώπου τόμος Α (Athens 1958).
2. Ἀραβαντινοῦ Α. Ἀσκληπιός καί Ἀσκληπιεία (Leipzig 1907).
3. Cure and Cult in Ancient Corinth. American School of Classical Studies at Athens (Princeton New Jersey 1977).
4. Παπαβασιλείου Ι, Ρόζου Β. Ἐγχειρίδιον, Ἱστορίας τῆς Ἰατρικῆς (Athens 1979).
5. Παυσανία Κορινθιακά.
6. Πουρναρόπουλου Γ. Ἱστορία τῆς Ἰατρικῆς διά μέσου τῶν αἰώνων (Athens 1952).
7. Ρόζου Β. Ἡ φυματίωσις παρ' Ἱπποκράτει καί Γαληνῷ (Athens 1973).
8. Τζάκου Κ. Ὀφθαλμολόγια τόμος Α (Athens 1954).
9. Τουλιάτου Δ. Ἡ Ἑλληνική Ἰατρική διά μέσου τῶν αἰώνων.
10. Χαραμῆ Ι. Χειρουργική τῶν Ὀφθαλμῶν (Athens 1954).

Address for correspondence: S. Chaviara-Karahaliou, Krokida 44, Kiaton, Greece.

Documenta Ophthalmologica **74**: 141–150, 1990.

King Sivi and Doctor Silv

M.V. VAN ANDEL
Meedenerweg 5, 9892 TB Feerwerd, The Netherlands

Abstract. The classical legend of ca. 500 BC about Buddha who in his former life as King Sivi wished to give a part of his body to the first one who asked for it, lies at the root of the success story of the indefatigable Dr Silva of Colombo, who succeeded through the oldest known story about donation of organs to make Sri Lanka the 'world champion' in eye donation. The legend is quoted in this article, followed by a short introduction of Dr Hudson Silva and his remarkable activities.

Sivi-Jātaka

Once upon a time, when the mighty King Sivi reigned in the city of Ariṭṭapura in the kingdom of Sivi, the Great Being[1] was born as his son. They called his name Prince Sivi. When he grew up, he went to Takkasilā and studied there; then returning, he proved his knowledge to his father the king, and by him was made viceroy. At his father's death he became king himself, and, forsaking the ways of evil, he kept the Ten Royal Virtues and ruled in righteousness. He caused six alms-halls to be built, at the four gates, in the midst of the city, and at his own door. He was munificent in distributing each day six hundred thousand pieces of money. On the eighth, fourteenth, and fifteenth days he never missed visiting the alms-halls to see the distribution made.

Once on the day of the full moon, the state umbrella had been uplifted early in the morning, and he sat on the royal throne thinking over the gifts he had given. Thought he to himself, 'Of all outside things there is nothing I have not given; But this kind of giving does not content me. I want to give something which is a part of myself. Well, this day when I go to the alms-hall, I vow that if anyone ask not something outside me, but name what is part of myself, – if he should mention my very heart, I will cut open my breast with a spear, and as though I were drawing up a water-lily, stalk and all, from a calm lake, I will pull forth my heart dripping with blood-clots and give it him: if he should name the flesh of my body, I will cut the flesh of my body and give it, as though I were graving with a graving tool: let him

[1] Name of Buddha.

142

name my blood, I will give him my blood, dropping it in his mouth or filling
a bowl with it: or again, if one say, I can't get my household work done,
come and do me a slave's part at home, then I will leave my royal dress and
stand without, proclaiming myself a slave, and slave's work I will do: should
any men demand my eyes, I will tear out my eyes and give them, as one
might take out the pith of a palm-tree.' Thus he thought within him:

"If there be any human gift that I have never made,
Be it my eyes, I'll give it now, all firm and unafraid."

Then he bathed himself with sixteen pitches of unperfumed water, and
adorned himself in all his magnificence, and after a meal of choice food he
mounted upon an elephant richly caparisoned and went to the alms-hall.

Sakka,[2] perceiving his resolution, thought: "King Sivi has determined to
give his eyes to any chance comer who may ask. Will you be able to do it,
or no?" He determined to try him; and, in the form of a brahmin[3] old and
blind, he posted himself on a high place, and when the king came to his
alms-hall he stretched out his hand and stood crying, "Long live the King!"
Then the king drove his elephant towards him, and said, "What do you say,
brahmin?" Sakka said to him, "O great king! in all the inhabited world there
is no spot where the fame of your munificent heart has not sounded. I am
blind, and you have two eyes." Then he asked for an eye:

"To ask an eye the old man comes from far, for I have none:
O give me one of yours, I pray, then we shall each have one."

When the Great Being heard this, thought he, 'Why that was just what I
was thinking in my palace before I came! What a fine chance! My heart's
desire will be fulfilled to-day; I shall give a gift which no man ever gave yet.'
And he recited the second stanza:

"Who taught thee hitherward to wend thy way,
O mendicant, and for an eye to pray?
The chiefest portion of a man is this,
And hard for men to part with, so they say."

"Sujampati among the gods, the same
Here among the men called Maghavā by name,

[2] King of the gods.
[3] Member of the class of priests.

He taught me hitherward to wend my way,
Begging and for an eye to urge my claim.

"'T is the all-chiefest gift for which I pray.
Give me an eye! O do not say me nay!
Give me an eye, that chiefest gift of gifts,
so hard for men to part with, as they say!"

"The wish that brought thee hitherward, the wish that did arise
Within thee, be that wish fulfilled. Here, brahmin, take my eyes.

"One eye thou didst request of me: behold, I give these two!
Go with good sight, in all the people's view;
so be thy wish fulfilled and now come true."

So much the king said. But, thinking it not meet that he should root out his eyes and bestow them there and then, he brought the brahmin indoors with him, and sitting on the royal throne, sent for a surgeon named Sīvaka. 'Take out my eye,' he then said.

Now all the city rang with the news, that the king wished to tear out his eyes and give them to a brahmin. Then the commander in chief, and all the other officials, and those beloved of the king, gathered together from the city and harem, and recited three stanzas, that they might turn the king from his purpose:

"O do not give thine eye, my lord; desert us not, O king!
Give money, pearls and coral give, and many a precious thing:

"Give thorobreds caparisoned, forth be the chariots rolled,
O king, drive up the elephants all fine with cloth of gold:

"These give, o king! that we may all preserve thee safe and sound,
Thy faithful people, with our cars and chariots ranged around."

Hereupon the king recited three stanzas:

"The soul which, having sworn to give, is then unfaithful found,
Puts his own neck within a snare low hidden on the ground.

"The soul which, having sworn to give, is then unfaithful found,
More sinful is than sin, and he to Yama's house[4] is bound.

"Unasked give nothing; neither give the thing he asketh not,

---

[4] I.e., hell.

144

This therefore which the brahmin asks, I give it on the spot."

Then the courtiers asked, "What do you desire in giving your eyes?" repeating a stanza:

"Life, beauty, joy, or strength – what is the prize,
O king, which motive for your deed supplies?
Why should the king of Sivi-land supreme
for the next world's sake thus give up his eyes?"

The king answered them in a stanza:

"In giving thus, not glory is my goal,
Not sons, not wealth, or kingdoms to control:
This is the good old way of holy men;
Of giving gifts enamoured is my soul."

To the Great Being's words the courtiers answered nothing; So the Great Being addressed Sīvaka the surgeon in a stanza:

"A friend and comrade, Sīvaka, art thou
Do as I bid thee – thou hast skill enow –
Take out my eyes, for this is my desire,
And in the beggar's hands bestow them now."

But Sīvaka said, "Bethink you, my lord! to give one's eyes is no light thing." – "Sīvaka, I have considered; don't delay, nor talk too much in my presence." Then he thought, "It is not fitting that a skillful surgeon like me should pierce a king's eyes with a lancet," so he pounded a number of simples, rubbed a blue lotus with the powder, and brushed it over the right eye: round rolled the eye, and there was great pain. "Reflect, my king, I can make it all right." – "Go on, friend, no delay, please." Again he rubbed in the powder, and brushed it over the eye: the eye started from the socket, the pain was worse than before. "Reflect, my king, I can still restore it." – "Be quick with the job!" A third time he smeared a sharper powder, and applied it: by the drug's power round went the eye, out came it from the socket, and hung dangling at the end of the tendon. "Reflect, my king, I can yet restore it again." – "Be quick." The pain was extreme, blood was trickling, the king's garments were stained with the blood. The king's women and courtiers fell at his feet, crying, "My lord, do not sacrifice your eyes!" loudly they wept and wailed. The king endured the pain, and said, "My friend, be

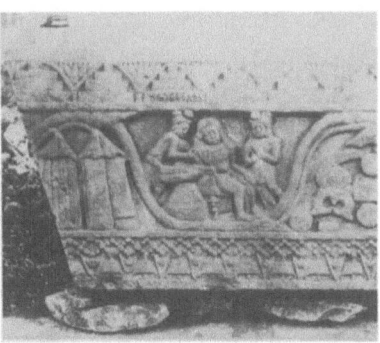

Fig. 1. The surgeon Sīvaka takes out Sivi's eyes. (Stupa of Bharhut, 2nd century Madhya Pradesh, India)

quick." "Very well, my lord," and the physician; and with his left hand grasping the eyeball took a knife in his right, and severing the tendon, laid the eye in the Great Being's hand, said, "Brahmin, come here." When the brahmin came near, he went on – "The eye of omniscience is dearer than this eye a hundredfold, aye a thousandfold: there you have my reason for this action," and he gave it to the brahmin, who raised it and placed it in his own eye socket. There it remained fixt by his power like a blue lotus in bloom. When the Great Being with his left eye saw that eye in his head, he cried – "Ah, how good is this my gift of an eye!" and thrilled straightway with the joy that had arisen within him, he gave the other eye also. Sakka placed this also in the place of his own eye, and departed from the king's palace, and then from the city, with the gaze of the multitude upon him, and went away to the multitude of gods.

In a short while the king's eyes began to grow; as they grew, and before they reached the top of the holes, a lump of flesh arose up inside like a ball of wool, filling the cavity; they were like doll's eyes, but the pain ceased. The Great Being remained in the palace a few days. Then he thought, "What has a blind man to do with ruling? I will hand over my kingdom to the courtiers, and go into my park, and become an ascetic, and live as a holy man." He summoned his courtiers, and told them what he intended to do. "One man," he said, "shall be with me, to wash my face, and so forth, and to do all that is proper, and you must fasten a cord to guide me to the retiring places." Then calling for his charioteer, he bade him to prepare the chariot. But the courtiers would not allow him to go in the chariot; they brought him out in a golden litter, and set him down by the lake side, and then, guarding him all around, returned. The king sat in the litter thinking of his gift.

At that moment Sakka's throne became hot; and he pondering perceived the reason. "I will offer the king a boon," thought he, "and make his eye well

146

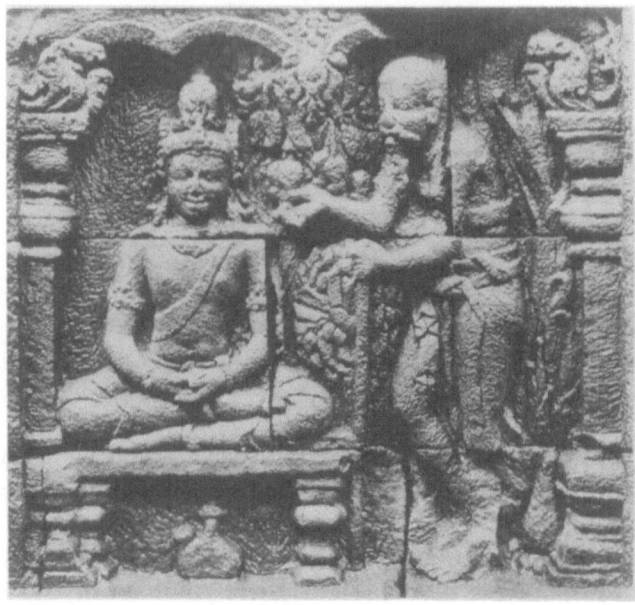

Fig. 2. Sakka disguised as a blind Brahmin with a stick asks the sitting King Sivi (Buddha in a former birth) for an eye (from: Beschrijving van de Barabudar; NJ Krom and T van Erp, 's Gravenhage 1920–1930)

again." So to that place he came; and not far off from the Great Being, he walked up and down, up and down.

"Who is that," cried the Great Being, when he heard the sound of the footsteps. Sakka repeated a stanza:

"Sakka, the king of gods, am I; to visit thee I came:
Choose thou a boon, O royal sage! whate'er thy wish may name."

The king replied with another stanza:

"Wealth, strength, and treasure without end, these I have left behind:
O Sakka, death and nothing more I want: for I am blind."

Then Sakka said, "Do you ask death, King Sivi, because you wish to die, or because you are blind?" – "Because I am blind, my lord." – "The gift is not everything in itself, your majesty, it is given with an eye to the future. Yet there is a motive relating to this visible world. Now you were asked for one eye, and gave two; make an Act of Truth about it." Then he began a stanza:

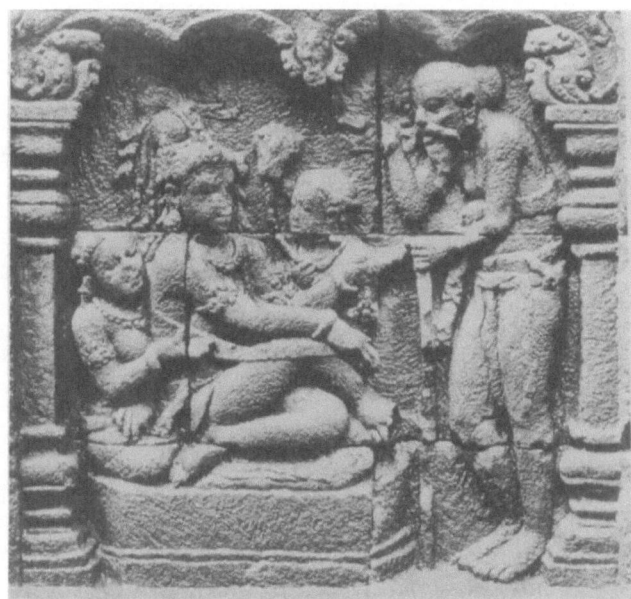

Fig. 3. King Sivi donates his eye, lying in the palm of his left hand to the blind Brahmin. In the middle the surgeon Sīvaka, with a lotus (?). (from: Beschrijving van de Barabudar; NJ Krom and T van Erp, 's Gravenhage 1920–1930)

"O warrior, lord of biped kind, declare the thing that's true:
If you the truth declare, your eye shall be restored to you."

On hearing this, the Great Being replied, "If you wish to give me an eye, Sakka, do not try another means, but let my eye be restored as a consequence of my gift." Sakka said, "Though they call me Sakka, king of the gods, your majesty, yet I cannot give an eye to anyone else; but the fruit of the gift by thee given, and by nothing else, your eye shall be restored to you." Then the other repeated a stanza, maintaining that his gift was well given:

"Whatever sort, whatever kind of suitor shall draw near,
Whoever comes to ask of me, he to my heart is dear:
If these my solemn words be true, now let my eye appear!"

Even as he uttered the words, one of his eyes grew up in the socket. Then he repeated a couple of stanzas to restore the other:

"A brahmin came to visit me, one of my eyes to crave:
Unto that brahmin mendicant the pair of them I gave.

148

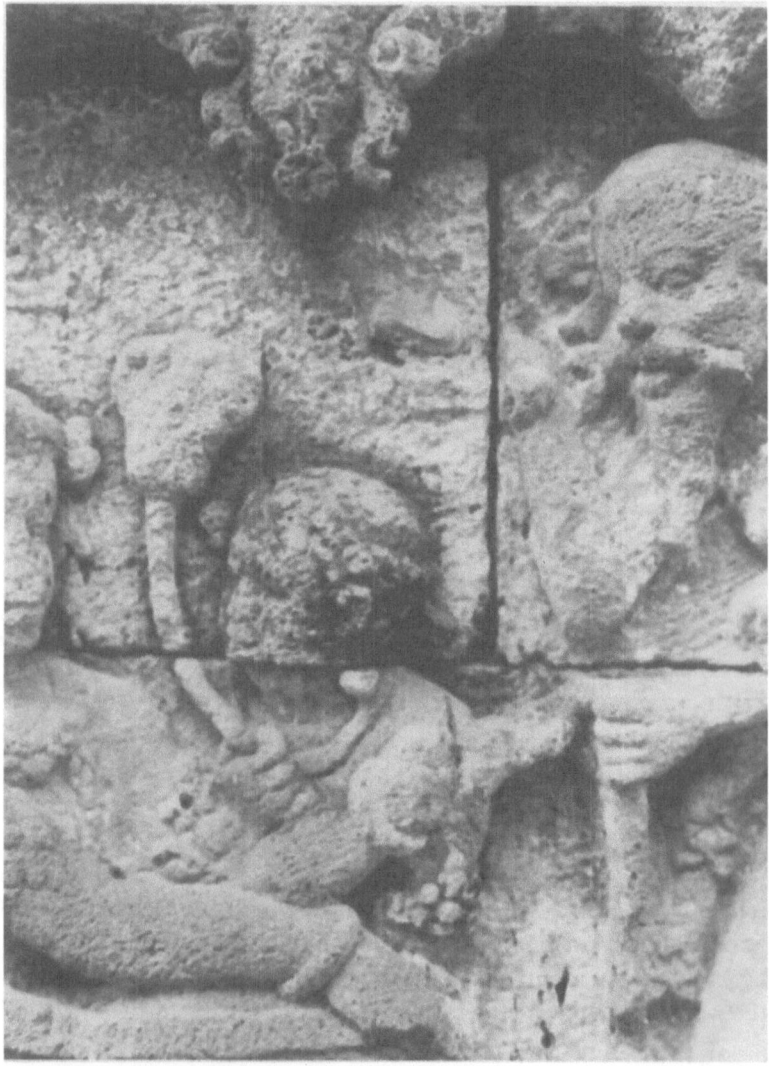

Fig. 4. Detail of the same relief sculpture, photographed some 60 years later. Relief much eroded (Borobudar; 800 AD. Central Java, Indonesia. Main entrance, first terrace, left hand, outside relief sculpture. Photograph, 1989, by PTVM de Jong, Rotterdam)

"A greater joy and more delight that action did afford.
If these my solemn words be true, be the other eye restored!"

On the instant appeared the second eye. But these eyes of his were neither natural nor divine. An eye given by Sakka as the brahmin, cannot be natural, we know; on the other hand, a divine eye cannot be produced in anything that is injured. But these eyes are called the eyes of Truth Absolute and Perfect. At that time when they came into existence, the whole royal retinue by Sakka's power was assembled; and Sakka standing in the midst of the throng, uttered praise in a couple of stanzas:

"O fostering king of Sililand, these holy hymns of thine
have gained for thee as bounty free this pair of eyes divine.

"Through rock and wall, o'er hill and dale, whatever bar may be,
A hundred leagues on every side those eyes of thine shall see."

Having uttered these stanzas, poised in the air before the multitude, with a last counsel to the Great Being that he should be vigilant, Sakka returned to the world of the gods. And the Great Being, surrounded by his retinue, went back in great pomp to the city, and entered the palace called Candaka, the Peacock's Eye. The news that he had got his eyes again spread abroad all through the Kingdom of Sivi. All the people gathered together to see him, with gifts in their hands. "Now all this multitude is come together," thought the Great Being, "I shall praise my gift that I gave." He caused a great pavilion to be put up at the palace gate, where he seated himself upon the royal throne, with the white umbrella spread above him. Then the drum was sent beating about the city, to collect all the trade guilds. Then he said, "O people of Sivi! now you have beheld these divine eyes, never eat food without giving something away!" and he repeated four stanzas, declaring the Law:

"Who, if he's asked to give, would answer no,
Although it be his best and choicest prize?
People of Sivi thronged in concourse, ho!
Come hither, see the gift of god, my eyes!

"Through rock and wall, o'er hill and dale, whatever bar may be,
A hundred leagues on every side these eyes of mine can see.

"Self-sacrifice in all men mortal living,
Of all things is most fine:
I sacrificed a mortal eye; and giving,
Received an eye divine.

"See, people! see, give ere ye eat, let others have a share.
This done with your best will and care,
Blameless to heaven you shall repair."

150

In these four verses he declared the Law; and after that, every fortnight, on the holy day, even every fifteenth day, he declared the Law in these same verses without cessation to a great gathering of people. Hearing which, the people gave alms and did good deeds, and went to swell the hosts of heaven.

Dr. Hudson Silva

Hudson Silva, a medical student in Colombo in 1957, decided to donate his eyes after he saw his first corneal transplantation. At that time the Ceylon Government had recently suspended the death penalty (traditionally, corneas were obtained mainly from executed prisoners). After graduation, Dr Silva started to write articles in the press, introducing the subject of eye donation as a meritorious service. In a Buddhistic temple he founded the Sri Lanka Eye Donation Society and soon he and his wife spoke in temples and during cremations, and laid funeral wreaths with ribbons on the graves of those people who donated their eyes. The Silva's are both devout Buddhists; they see the bequest of eyes not only as a good deed but also as a pious duty.

The enucleation is done openly without medical or professional secrecy. It is tradition that the relatives look on with attention and respect when the eyes are removed. The relatives are always informed about the name of the recipients. The publication of the list of donors and recipients stimulate potential donors. The call for eyes was so successful that already in 1963 there were signs of a surplus of eyes, so Dr Silva started the following year to export eyes to various countries of Asia. Until June 1989, 25,000 eyes have been donated to 135 eye centres in 54 countries. The eye bank is now manned 24 hours a day with 13 coworkers paid for by non-governmental donations. About one third of the total Sri Lanka export nowadays goes to Pakistan.

Last year, Dr Hudson Silva received a 'doctor honoris causa' degree of Groningen University, The Netherlands, 'to honour the impressive way in which he and Mrs Silva inspired and provided leadership in the human aspects of the medical sciences'.

Reference

1. The JĀKATA or stories of Buddha's former births from the Pali by various hands. Vol. IV, p. 250–256, Cowell & Rouse, University Press, Cambridge 1901

Address for offprints: Dr M.V. van Andel, Meedenerweg 5, 9892 TB Feerwerd, The Netherlands.

HISTORY OF OPHTHALMOLOGY 1

CONTENTS

KLUWER ACADEMIC PUBLISHERS   ACOI 1   ISBN 0-89838-366-8

HISTORY OF OPHTHALMOLOGY 2

CONTENTS

KLUWER ACADEMIC PUBLISHERS   ACOI 2   ISBN 0-7923-0273-7

A History of Surgery

With Emphasis on the Netherlands

by **Dr D. De Moulin**

After a career as an active surgeon, the author
of this volume switched to medical history and
he is now Professor of the History of Medicine
at the Catholic University, Nijmegen, The Netherlands. Professor De Moulin is also author
of a previous publication, A Short History of
Breast Cancer' (Martinus Nijhoff Publishers),
which has gained world-wide attention.
A History of Surgery consists of original research into the development of surgery through
the ages and provides a chronological survey
of the events which have led to the modern
achievements in surgery. Furthermore, the
book contains many historical illustrations not
previously published.
There is an emphasis on surgical practice
within the Netherlands. Dutch surgery, however, has by no means been taken as an isolated
phenomenon: it is considered in its context
within European Surgery as a whole, whilst
contemporary medical thinking is set against
a cultural and political background.
As a result of this unique approach, this volume
will be of great interest to practicing surgeons
and physicians, as well as to medical historians
and the public at large.

Highlight

Contents
1. The Roots of Western Surgery. **2.** The Western Middle Ages. **3.** The Renaissance. **4.** The
Golden Age. **5.** The Age of Enlightenment.
6. Practical Surgery in the 17th and 18th Centuries. **7.** The Beginning of Modern Surgery.
8. Antisepsis: A Turning Point in Surgery. **9.** The
German Period in Dutch Surgery. **10.** Surgery
in the Past 75 Years. References. Bibliography.
Index.

**KLUWER
ACADEMIC
PUBLISHERS**

1987, 432 pp.   ISBN 0-89838-968-2
Hardbound Dfl. 251.00/£83.75/US$101.00

P.O. Box 322, 3300 AH Dordrecht, The Netherlands
P.O. Box 358, Accord Station, Hingham, MA 02018-0358, U.S.A.